A DENTAL PRACTI
SERIES EDITED BY DONALD

PREVENTIVE DENTISTRY

JOHN O. FORREST
FDS RCS (Eng), FICD

*Formerly of the Department of Periodontology
and Preventive Dentistry, Guy's Hospital
Formerly Senior Hospital Dental Officer in Charge of the School of
Dental Hygiene, Guy's Hospital, London*

Second Edition

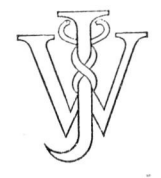

BRISTOL: JOHN WRIGHT & SONS LTD
1981

© J. O. Forrest, 6 Harcourt House, 19A Cavendish Square, London, W1M 9AD
1981

All Rights Reserved. No part of this publication may be reproduced, stored in a retrieval system, or transmitted in any form or by any means, electronic, mechanical, photocopying, recording or otherwise, without the prior permission of the copyright owner.

Published by John Wright & Sons Ltd, 42–44 Triangle West, Bristol, BS8 1EX

First edition, 1976
Second edition, 1981

British Library Cataloguing in Publication Data

Forrest, John Orchover
Preventive dentistry. — 2nd ed.
— (A 'Dental practitioner' handbook; no. 22)
1. Preventive dentistry
I. Title   II. Series
617.6'01   RK60.7

ISBN 0 7236 0553 X

PRINTED IN GREAT BRITAIN BY HENRY LING LTD, A SUBSIDIARY OF
JOHN WRIGHT & SONS LTD, AT THE DORSET PRESS, DORCHESTER, DT1 1HD

PREFACE TO THE SECOND EDITION

THE AIM of the first edition of this book was to show that preventive dentistry can be made to work successfully in practice. Emphasis was placed on simplicity and in general the absence of special gadgets, gimmickry and costly procedures. However, because it was an *introduction* to preventive dentistry the text largely dealt with techniques and materials which had proved successful over the years for the majority of patients. It was, however, too easy to dismiss the minority of failures as 'unteachable' and to hope that eventually they would 'go away'.

In recent years there has been a surprising and gratifying adoption on the part of many practices of preventive methods and combined with outside influences, such as the almost universal use of fluoride dentifrices, we are seeing a considerable improvement in oral health.

The majority of dental schools (regrettably, not all) have begun to emphasize the preventive attitude and many new graduates are setting up purposely designed premises where they can practise dentistry based on a preventive basis. The fact that they are beginning to find this financially rewarding as well is an answer to those who over the years questioned whether reducing the load of repair dentistry could bring about a reduction in income.

A stage has now been reached when there should be a pause for assessment of our results and we should question whether our attitudes (not necessarily techniques) need to be modified in order to achieve further progress. *Knowing* what must be done is not necessarily going to bring a successful result if much of the responsibility is to be placed with the patient. Although the goal is the continuing oral health of the community we must be conscious of the fact that we are dealing with non-lethal diseases and hence motivation in the young by fear of the future consequences of neglect is not easy. This is of course true in other areas of medicine dealing with potential high risks and examples can be quoted of the continuation of cigarette smoking by large sections of the population, the neglect of seat belt use, the ingestion of harmful foods and drink, and the increase in the use of the 'hard' drugs.

Thus attention has been given to assessment and motivation of the individual patient rather than as previously merely as an inducement

PREFACE TO THE SECOND EDITION

to brush and floss. More attention must be paid to improving the success rate in the teaching of home oral care on a long term basis. Therefore we must avoid complacency at apparent success which may be short term and bring back the patient for repeated regular 'refreshers'.

Some of the materials previously mentioned or recommended are no longer available and some have been replaced by new and modified types. Where possible these have been included, and reference has been made to the preventive role which can be played by restorative materials. Other chapters and sections have been rewritten, it is hoped with a more up-to-date text. The changes in most areas of dentistry in so short a time are quite remarkable and no doubt much of this will have been outmoded almost by the time of publication. In particular the chapter 'The Child Patient' has been expanded to include the expectant mother and the newly born child.

It is disappointing that the most important positive preventive procedure that does not depend on patient co-operation, i.e. fluoridation of water supplies has made little progress in implementation in recent years, certainly in the U.K. In fact, because of the well organized opposition there are probably some fewer areas receiving optimally fluoridated water than say five years ago. This must be of concern to all of us who are interested in effecting the oral health of the community for minimum cost. To discuss ways and means of influencing the responsible bodies is unfortunately beyond the scope of this book, but every member of the dental team must be aware of its importance and perhaps try to influence his or her own colleagues and local authorities for its adoption. It would seem now that perhaps this propaganda is best carried out on an individual, not organized basis. In spite of this the future of preventive dentistry looks brighter than ever and if carried on with the same enthusiasm as in the last ten years, the next decade will see a marked diminution in the amount of dental destruction, but more important, an eventual large increase of the period of tooth retention. In view of the very adequate publication *Fluorides in Caries Prevention* by John J. Murray (*Dental Practitioner Handbook No. 20*) which is a series companion to this text, little detailed discussion of fluorides has been entered into here. Fuller explanations are given by Professor Murray.

J. O. F.

PREFACE TO THE FIRST EDITION

THERE must be very cogent reasons for yet another book on preventive dentistry. Every intending author should be asked, or should ask himself, why he is going to all that trouble? His reply ought to be: 'Because what I have to say hasn't been said before, or not in the way I want to say it.' I have been distressed (but not wholly surprised) at the present trend in many published works dealing with prevention. The attitude seems to be one of replacement of the dentist's traditional mechanical restorative role by mechanical and laboratory preventive devices and a 'philosophy' which bids to replace the patient's hitherto enormous expenditure on full mouth rehabilitation by enormous expenditure on a full 'preventive control programme'. We have a new (costly) terminology that has developed and there is talk of the ministrations of such exotic flowers as 'disease control therapists' or 'disease control receptionists'. The 'new' discovery of 'plaque' has been hailed as something like the first landing on the moon. It is rarely mentioned that dentists have been dealing with plaque and practising successful preventive dentistry throughout this century (and before), without the gimmickry, special gadgets, audiovisual rooms, high sounding terminology, and hence with very little expense to the patient except for cost of the dentist's time. The tools he used and should still use are dedication, care, continuing evaluation of his long-standing patients, and above all a burning enthusiasm and a belief in the value of his work. In the current enthusiasm for plaque control there seems to be some belief that careful scaling is no longer required!

The attempt here is to show what works successfully in practice—evaluated over 27 years—and above all what works simply, inexpensively and with a minimum of gimmickry and ballyhoo.

The author's sincere thanks are due to Mr. H. Colin Davis and Professor A. H. R. Rowe for reading the manuscript and offering helpful suggestions. I am grateful to Professor W. J. Tulley for his help with regard to aspects of preventive orthodontics in Chapter 6 and to Mr. Jeffrey Rose for the information given in the same chapter. I would like to thank Mrs. Eileen Jaffe for kindly providing the illustrations for *Fig.* 34 and Mr. David Boxall for *Figs.* 35, 36 and 37.

PREFACE TO THE FIRST EDITION

I should like to express my thanks to Dr. Donald Derrick who invited me to produce this Handbook and never became exasperated at missed deadlines, and to Mr. A. N. Boyd and Mr. G. A. Moore of John Wright & Sons Ltd who proved to be so helpful at the production stage.

Finally, I wish to pay a tribute to Dr. G. H. Leatherman for encouraging my fledgeling interest in real preventive dentistry all those years ago in the R.A.F.

J. O. F.

CONTENTS

Foreword	ix
1. The Change to Preventive Dentistry	1
2. Examination, Diagnosis, Patient Assessment and Treatment Planning	9
3. Dental Plaque and its Control	19
4. Control of the Common Dental Diseases Part 1. Prevention of Caries	57
5. Control of the Common Dental Diseases Part 2. Periodontal Disease	72
6. The Mother and Child	90
7. Preventive Aspects of Restorative Dentistry	110
8. Preventive Dentistry and Sports Activities	116
Appendix 1. Materials for use in the Preventive Practice	120
Appendix 2. Summary of Procedure for Prevention of Caries and Periodontal Disease	124
Appendix 3. Some Practical Problems	126
Index	127

FOREWORD

Maury Massler DDS, MS, DSc
Department of Restorative Dentistry, Tufts University, Boston, Massachusetts

IN this book the topic of *Preventive Dentistry* is approached in a very honest and practical fashion. It is written in a lucid and attractive style. This is a refreshing contrast to the heavily detailed textbooks which rest on our shelves as 'reference texts' but to which we seldom refer.

It should be read by every senior dental student as an introduction to the *modern* practice of dentistry. It should be read by their teachers, and quoted frequently to bring into focus the true objective of a dental education and practice—the *prevention* of oral and dental diseases concomitant with the surgical repair of these diseases when prevention fails, as so often occurs. The practising dentist (general practitioner and specialist), to whom this book is directed, should read it as a review of 'where we are and what we must do' in the art and science of *Preventive Dentistry*.

In making his excellent evaluation of the large number of articles on *Preventive Dentistry* to be found in almost every publication, Mr. Forrest saves us many hours of perusal of the current literature on prevention.

CHAPTER 1

THE CHANGE TO PREVENTIVE DENTISTRY

WHEREAS previously a trend toward the implementation of preventive methods in dental practice was just discernible, the most recent years have in fact demonstrated a most noticeable change in the attitude and acceptance by the profession and public of the importance of primary care as an integral part of total dentistry.

This has to be considered from two aspects; in respect of the community as a whole and as applied to the individual patient/dentist relationship. Leatherman (1979) states, 'At present more than half the world's population do not have the benefit of a primary health care service.' He quotes the World Health Organisation (1978) definition as follows, 'Primary health care is essential health care made universally accessible to individuals and families in the community by means acceptable to them, through their full participation and at a cost the community and country can afford. It forms an integral part both of the country's health system of which it is the nucleus and of the overall social and economic development of the community.' He goes on to state, 'It is the dental profession's responsibility to teach and motivate whole communities to carry out daily preventive dental health routines and to cooperate by becoming involved in the planning, operation and control of primary dental health care services. It is perhaps worthy of note that there is the possibility that the dental profession has developed such an efficient replacement service to the individual, that it has discouraged patient demand for effective preventive and restorative service. Nor is prevention encouraged by the design of many health programmes.'

While it is beyond the scope of this book to describe the community aspects of primary health care, the dentist in practice will undoubtedly benefit from any improvements in the general standard of oral health in the community by reduction in his work load and by the creation of a group of patients who are more likely to be educated to accept his individual teaching.

When considering the ravages of caries, preventive dentistry should begin with water fluoridation of the community drinking water which is inexpensive and requires no patient cooperation. White (1975) says, 'Most of the methods rely on some form of patient cooperation and generally cost much more than fluoridation of the communal water supply. The central task in making these other methods effective is to gain the cooperation of the patient.

To accomplish this it is important that the dentist understands the interests of the patient, not that the patient understands the interests of the dentist.' He goes on to say, 'Comprehensive fast teaching programs—including lengthy verbal explanations, brochures, pamphlets, film strips and movies—should not be relied on as an important means of patient education. How many carious lesions have these procedures stopped from occurring?' Indeed the need for caution in our claims for preventive public health measures is stressed by Horowitz (1977) '... dental health programs, including expensive "plaque control programs", have been billed as a panacea for oral health. Dental health education in schools, including teaching oral hygiene procedures, has not been shown to prevent tooth decay.... If oral hygiene procedures are to be introduced in schools, they should be recognized for their known value of reducing gingivitis, and then only when the procedures are supervised'.

What is in fact happening today is that dental practice is taking the following form:

1. There are many dentists who believe wholly in prevention in all its forms, in research, teaching and lecturing to the profession and to the public, and clinically applying methods to put their convictions into practice.
2. Other dentists—at present the majority—feel that their training has equipped them to treat the considerable amount of existing dental disease, and will continue to do this to increasingly higher standards using more and more ancillary help.
3. Ideally an ever-growing number of dentists are combining the attitudes 1 and 2 above, and practise a modified approach by maintaining a preventive attitude to all the restorative and other forms of dentistry which are planned, and by simultaneously influencing the patient in a like manner.

The following are some of the major factors influencing the dentists' attitude toward preventive dentistry:

1. Although for years dentists were aware that much of their work, however expertly and carefully carried out, was liable to break down in many mouths, with recurrent caries or loss of abutments of complex and expensive bridgework through periodontal disease, they attributed this on the whole to faults in their materials or methods. That these faults—imperfect filling materials, difficulties in tooth preparation, etc.—existed is not denied, but when methods and materials became even more sophisticated and breakdown of work continued, some dentists became concerned that something more needed to be done. With the advent of the air turbine handpiece, cavity and tooth preparation became so simplified that tooth

substance was removed in a wholesale (and sometimes indiscriminate) fashion. Much of this work has adhered to Black's principles of cavity preparation with extension for prevention, often taken to its limits of full coverage. And yet recurrent caries still occurred. The more treatment was given the more breakdown occurred, except in a fortunate few.

2. As modern dentistry became technically more sophisticated it also became more expensive and patients themselves complained about further extensive work which was required so soon after previous considerable expenditure.

3. The public was made aware of research into preventive aspects of dentistry often reported in news media with little basis on immediate fact (e.g. the furore over dextranase). Magazines and TV programmes featured preventive methods as less uncomfortable than conventional drilling. A demand for these methods has come from the public and this too has partly influenced dentists.

4. One's own experience with preventive dentistry lectures and courses indicates that the main interest has come from young dentists with about 5 years' practice history. At about this time their dissatisfaction with the results of their work reaches a peak and even if preventive methods had not existed they would have turned to some other alternative to the daily soul destroying method of earning a livelihood by 'amalgam pushing'.

There is now a further generation of young dentists who have been trained and indoctrinated in the dental schools by inspired teachers and believe in preventive dentistry as total practice. These graduates are setting up practices designed with prevention as their main objective. The response from the public has been startling and gratifying (Lewis et al., 1979).

Discouragement to change may be based on the following:

1. In the U.K. under the terms of the National Health Service, and possibly under other third party payment schemes, there is no encouragement of preventive methods in dentistry. At least, this is the belief of the majority of dentists. It must, however, be a matter of disappointment that a dentist can receive repeated fees for filling the same tooth at regular intervals but no fee for a topical fluoride.

2. The dentist is uncertain which of the many advertised products he should use. The claims may be conflicting. He is worried that some of the recommended materials and appliances are now very expensive.

3. There is uncertainty on how to explain the practice change to the patient.

4. An important question arises. If the amount of restorative

work is cut down what happens to his income? (A question which in many recent reports appears to have been answered satisfactorily.)

The dentist is not yet convinced, because he has seen few long-term clinical results, that prevention really works. He is struggling with his basic training in 'scorched earth dentistry' which taught him only to cut out or destroy faulty areas.

Thus the following chapters will be devoted to resolving these doubts and explaining how the practice can make a successful change to prevention. But no text can inspire the same enthusiasm as the eventual chairside clinical evaluation of the effects of caring for health rather than treating already established disease.

Many of the techniques which are applied in preventive dentistry particularly with regard to caries control and periodontal disease are carried out by the dental hygienist and they are trained not only to do this but to give support by teaching home care and giving advice to patients about diet control and growth, etc. Very considerable detail of this kind will be found in the textbooks devoted to the teaching of hygienists such as Wilkins (1976) and Collins et al. (1978).

THE PHILOSOPHY OF CHANGE TO PREVENTION IN THE DENTAL PRACTICE

It has been stated in the foregoing that many dentists are eager to make the change from purely repair dentistry to one which considers prevention as a first priority. It should be stressed to those who may still consider that it is possible to catch up with the growing dental disease problem by expanding the number of available dentists that the results of other countries have shown that this does not work. We may take as an example Sweden, where the problem of a surplus of dentists was becoming manifest (S.O.U. 1970) but still the rate of dental destruction continued to increase. Many authorities in other countries have, however come to realize that the so-called lack of dentists is not entirely responsible for the failure to halt the progression of dental disease. Indeed, one factor must be that as restorative dentistry becomes more highly developed treatment becomes restricted to fewer patients because of the increased time taken, and of course the considerable cost. As stated by Jacobson (1972), 'Highly developed dentistry creates a "vicious circle" of increasing need for dental treatment'. It must be concluded that on the whole our existing dental manpower has been misused and it becomes necessary to foster and encourage a change of attitude on the part of both the dentist and the patient.

THE ATTITUDE OF THE DENTIST

1. The dentist must be confident that preventive methods really work and must hence resist the constant temptation to follow his early basic training which conditions him to drill out the sticky fissure as a so-called 'preventive measure'.

2. Thus the essential factor in the prevention of caries is to *resist* drilling teeth unless this is completely unavoidable. The investigation of pits and fissures with a very sharp pointed probe followed by the bur where the probe *just* sticks is not good preventive dentistry. It often results in the patient possessing teeth which may be 'peppered' with small amalgam fillings and as Phillips (1965) and Going (1972) have shown all fillings are susceptible to leakage. The

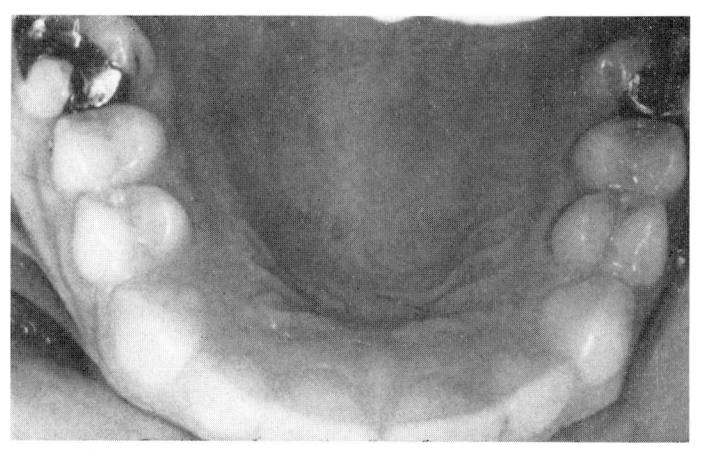

Fig. 1. The first molars were filled with amalgam but subsequently topical fluorides were applied regularly. The remaining teeth are sound but the filled teeth require further attention.

incipient caries in sticky pits and fissures (if indeed it *is* caries) will usually respond to repeated topical applications of fluoride solutions —and this is true whether the incipient breach of surface is on the proximal surface or on the occlusal. (*Figs.* 1–3.)

3. Prevention is a team undertaking. It cannot be carried out in isolation by a single member of that team. Everyone connected with the care of the patient must be aware of the necessity for working within a framework of promoting health first in all procedures carried out.

4. The dentist must believe, and show that he believes, that prevention really works. If he reveals uncertainty and lack of confidence he will be unable to influence his patients sufficiently for them to adopt the new attitude to dental health.

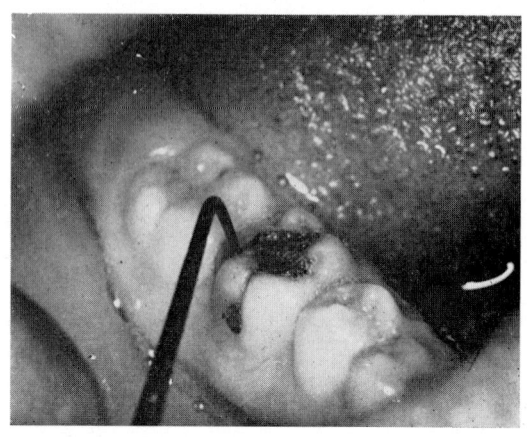

Fig. 2. The repaired part of the tooth is most vulnerable even if the restoration is better finished than here.

5. The whole practice, all the staff—ancillaries, secretary receptionist (and also technicians), must feel this same confidence radiating from the dentist. Many hygienists, for example, are regrettably trained as scaling technicians and have not had the opportunity at training school because of the shortness of the course to see the

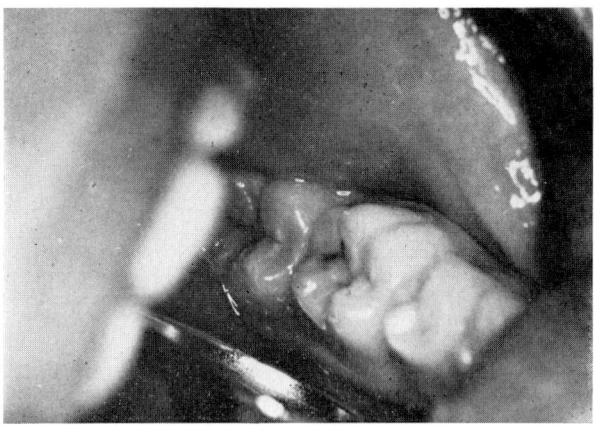

Fig. 3. Pits and fissures treated with stannous fluoride become brown and hard. No drilling is necessary.

long-term effects of preventive methods. Therefore it is often necessary for the attitude of such hygienists to be changed to a less technically and more preventively-orientated one. We must also consider the patient to be a member of the dental team because of the importance of patient co-operation.

One possible reason why the preventive approach has not been entirely successful to date is that dentists formulated a policy of prevention and expected all patients to conform to a pattern of learning which was fairly rigid. We should study the behaviour pattern of each patient and modify our plans as the relationship changes. Thus we should make individual assessments as to each patient's need for special care, e.g. fluoride application, plaque control, dietary counselling, according to their susceptibility to breakdown. In addition, we should give special consideration and careful prognosis to the patient with an apparently healthy mouth, but with some problematic systemic condition.

It may be that we should be giving more emphasis to the immediate virtues of positive health than threatening the dire effects of a disease which to the young may be too far ahead to be of much concern.

6. Prevention is a continuous process. It does not end with training of the patient at the first few visits but will continue throughout the practice life of the patient in the form of careful reappraisal of the patient's dental health control practice and the resulting oral state.

7. The dentist must be convinced that prevention does not consist of technical procedures. Neither is it a question of which fluoride, which fissure sealant or which kind of floss to use. This approach is a result of the reluctance to reject the mechanical approach bred into the dentist and also of the assumed desire of the patient (or the fee-paying agent) to receive something tangible and visible for the fee charged. It is the author's own belief that the present use of fissure sealants comes into this category. In a sense fissure sealants are currently for those who do not yet really believe in total preventive dentistry.

8. Preventive methods should be easy to carry out for both the dentist (or dental team) and, especially, for the patient.

9. Methods and techniques which are expensive either because of the time taken or because of the high cost of materials should not be considered as acceptable. This is a further argument against such materials as fissure sealants (*see* 7 *above*).

10. It is all too easy to believe that preventive dentistry is synonymous with caries prevention. In fact periodontal disease is responsible for a greater tooth loss and is often ignored until too late. And yet in the early stages gingivitis and periodontal disease are readily controlled and reversible.

11. We should consider whether it is always necessary to 'do something' for any deviation from what we consider or have been taught is 'normal'. Thus in addition to 'sticky fissures' in (1) above should we *always* eliminate or treat occlusal discrepancies, attrition, or periodontal pockets deeper than an optimum measurement?

12. Finally, and most important, prevention does not consist in placing one's patients indiscriminately on rigid plaque control programmes; it does not consist in sending them into an audiovisual room to look at pictures and posters. The conscience of the dentist should not be satisfied by presenting the patient with a bag of preventive aids containing toothbrush, dentifrice, floss, disclosing tablets, wood points, interspace brush and a pamphlet of instructions.

REFERENCES

Collins W. J. N., Forrest J. O. and Walsh T. F. (1978) *A Handbook for Dental Hygienists*. Bristol, Wright.
Going R. E. (1972) Microleakage around dental restorations: A summarising review. *J. Am. Dent. Assoc.* **84,** 1349.
Horowitz A. M. (1977) Editorial. *J. Public Health Dent.* **37,** 4.
Jacobson L. (1972) Training and utilization of dental personnel. *Oral Hygiene*. Copenhagen, Munksgaard p. 106.
Leatherman G. H. (1979) A primary preventive dental service. *Br. Dent. J.* **147,** 167.
Lewis K. J., Taylor J. A., McCann C. J. et al. (1979) The delivery of practical prevention in general practice. *Dent. Practice* 17/3 12–19.
Phillips R. W. (1965) Cavity varnishes and bases. *Dent. Clin. North Am.* March, 159–168.
Statens Offentliga Utredningar (1970) Swedish Dental Health Service: Expansion and Organization. *Sver. Tandläk Forb. Tidn.* **11,** 38.
White G. E. (1975) *Dental Caries: A Multifactorial Disease*. Springfield Ill., Thomas.
Wilkins E. M. (1976) *Clinical Practice of the Dental Hygienist*, Philadelphia, Lea & Febiger.

CHAPTER 2

EXAMINATION, DIAGNOSIS, PATIENT ASSESSMENT AND TREATMENT PLANNING

WE should be aware of the different stages of prevention as relating to the approach to disease control:
1. Primary Prevention: Steps taken to ensure that disease does not occur.
2. Secondary Prevention: Detection of incipient disease and halting its progression by simple repair or remedial measures. Sometimes at this stage there may be 'reversal' to the normal (as in gingivitis).
3. Tertiary Prevention: Treatment of well established disease in order to minimize or eliminate the gross destructive effects, to restore healthy function and to resist further attacks of the disease process.

Dentists have in general started their disease control at stage 2 above. Their training equipped them to search carefully for early caries, and dealing with this was thought to be the best approach possible. The result was a mouth with numerous small fillings in the pits and fissures. At stage 3 above or later the presence of periodontal disease was noted but all too often this awareness came too late.

THE ORAL MUCOSA

Caries and periodontal disease are not the only disorders for which dentists should be searching. The dentist should be on the alert for more potentially serious diseases, especially of the oral mucosa. The report on *Oral Cancer in England and Wales* (Binnie et al., 1972) gives the number of deaths from intra-oral cancer as 60 per cent of registrations. This is largely put down to the predominance of late stage disease at the start of treatment. The authors question how adequately the dentist carries out his important function of early diagnosis. They imply that there is limitation of diagnosis by limitation of training.

Binnie (1976) states that from 1960 to 1970 both lip and oral cancer in men (in the U.K.), but not women, have been steadily decreasing. He speculates that there may be some link between the decrease in oral cancer with an improvement in oral hygiene. He also states that there would appear to be a positive correlation between pipe and cigar smoking and oral cancer, but a negative one with cigarette smoking and therefore the known decrease in non-cigarette tobacco consumption might appear to have some influence.

The clinical examination has hitherto been a hard tissue examination: cavities are noted and often the drilling is started at the same visit. In order to overcome the 'conditioning' given to dentists during training, the hard tissues should be examined *last*, the survey thus starting at the neck, where the lymph nodes are palpated for enlargement and hardening, and then lips, cheeks, tongue, palate are viewed and if necessary palpated. Any abnormality should be carefully noted and the extent of any lesion should be measured and recorded.

THE PREVENTIVE APPROACH IN TREATMENT PLANNING

Before embarking on any course of restorative treatment, our first aim should be the maintenance or achievement of the oral health of the patient. At the same time we should also be concerned with the patient's general sense of wellbeing, which should if possible be improved. Our approach should therefore be along the following lines:

1. Establishment of communication between the dentist and patient.
2. History taking: general; dental.
3. Clinical examination.
4. Use of diagnostic aids.
5. Preliminary planning discussion with patient.
6. Initial preparation by a member of the dental team (and this to include personal care and training).
7. Reassessment.
8. Discussion of definitive plan.
9. Final treatment to be carried out (if any).

If we examine each of these points we can establish a set of conditions as a guide for relating dental treatment to each case as it presents.

1. *Communication*

It is necessary from the outset to listen to the patient who has originally presented with some idea of what she or he *wants*. This is the reason for coming to the dentist. It may be to restore an anterior incisor. It may not coincide with our own later estimate of the 'ideal' programme for this patient. It is also necessary for the dentist to introduce at this stage, i.e. as early as possible, the idea that the attitude of the practice is 'different'. It is one of prevention. This may be explained to the patient by a number of analogies, e.g.

DIAGNOSIS AND TREATMENT PLANNING

filling teeth without practising preventive methods is like putting new windows in a burning house.

2. *History Taking*

Usually taken in two parts: *General* (medical) history, past and present; *Dental* history, past and present.

It is logical to check on the patient's medical background first and having recorded any relevant facts to follow up with an enquiry as to past and present dental disorders and any treatment carried out. Sometimes it may be expedient to listen to the 'dental story' first, especially if the patient is attending because of pain or other emergency, and follow up with the medical history.

A careful record must be made of any medications which the patient admits to taking. The question should not be phrased, 'Are you taking any drugs?' or words to that effect. The meaning to many is, 'Are you an addict?' It is better to ask, 'Are you using any medicaments?' This widens the question from oral or parenteral intake, to cover skin application. This may give a clue to skin lesions which leads to greater awareness of possible related oral mucosa conditions.

Any important aspects should be clearly marked and attention should be drawn on the 'work chart' to any special disorders requiring care. This is always effected in practice by sticking a self-adhesive red star to the top right of the chart—beside it the condition requiring caution, e.g. 'Rheumatic fever *x* years ago' (*Fig.* 4).

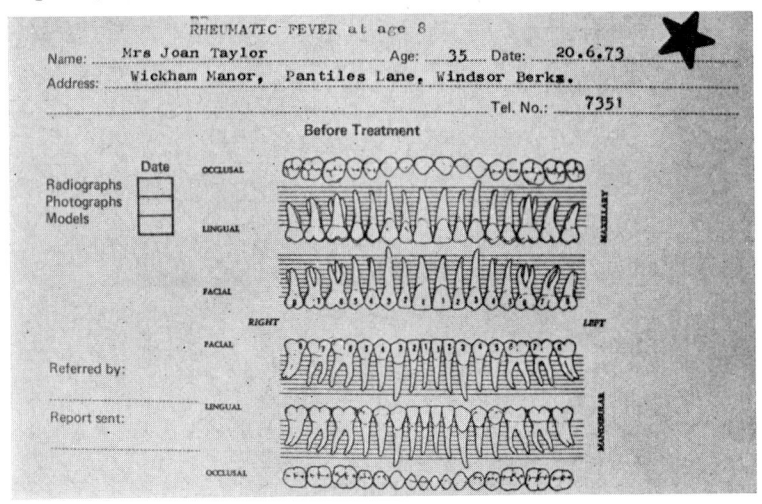

Fig. 4. Dental chart with warning signal (red) in top right corner. This indicates that special care is necessary because of some unusual condition, which is noted briefly on top of the chart but fully in the patient's medical history.

Complaints of oral pain are recorded as requiring urgent attention.

At this stage by listening to the patient it will be possible to discover personality problems, perhaps by hearing accounts of the patient's experiences with other (unnamed) dentists and, most important, an estimation of the 'dental I.Q.' can be made. This is a measure of the patient's ability to comprehend the facts about his dental condition and his keenness to be involved in any discussion of treatment planning.

3. *Clinical Examination*

Before commencing, the dentist should be confident of his ability to see clearly and distinctly all those areas of the mouth and jaws which he will be assessing. This depends on there being a sufficient level of lighting and also on his own visual acuity. The ability to focus at close range becomes more difficult with the ageing process, and the use of aids to vision such as loupes or telescopes is highly recommended. The best ones are custom-made to the wearer's own prescription. Probably the most comfortable and useful are those supplied by 'Designs for Vision' (*Fig.* 5) (*see* Appendix 1).

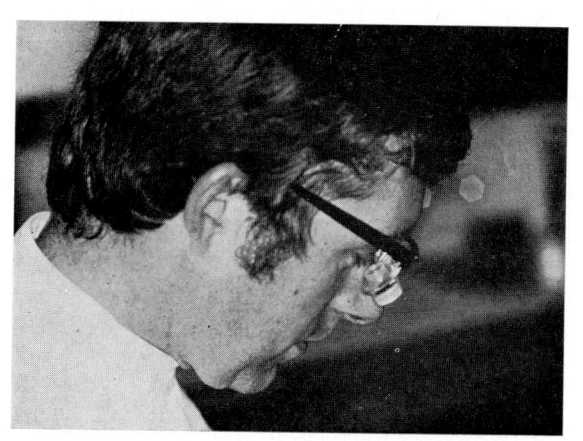

Fig. 5. Use of custom-made telescopes to wearer's own prescription.

There should be an examination of the whole person, not rows of teeth. It starts as the patient walks through the door and sits in the chair. Signs of weakness, nervousness, facial pallor, cyanosis of lips, exophthalmos, breathlessness etc. should be noted.

Following the history taking and discussion, the patient, who is comfortably seated, is asked to close the mouth (every patient automatically opens the mouth when approached by a dentist), and the face, head and neck are carefully inspected in the mouth-closed position, and any apparent abnormalities are recorded. Following this the patient is asked to open the lips keeping the teeth in occlusion and a careful inspection is made of the entire vestibular surface of the lips, cheek, gingivae and teeth. The patient is asked to open and close the jaws in centric, and any deviation of the mandible on opening is noted. During closing movements of the mandible it is

a

b

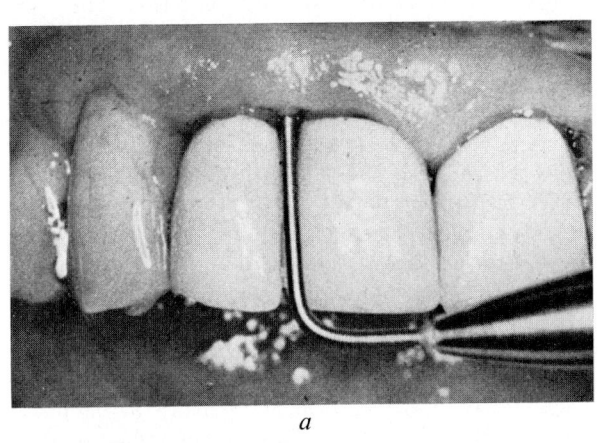

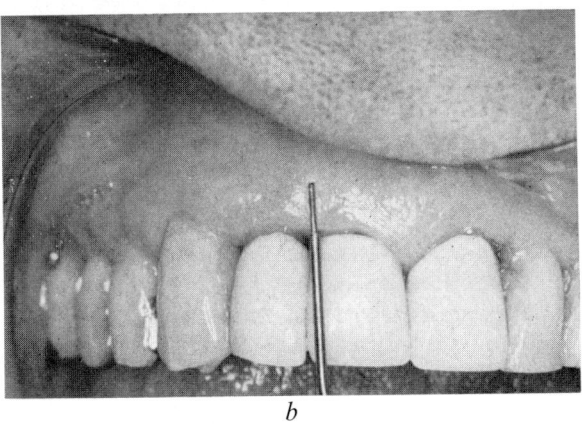

Fig. 6. *a*, End of periodontal probe deep in pocket. *b*, Probe on outside of gum showing depth. The exact measurement can be read on the sliding handle (Svenska Dentomax).

important to look for cuspal interference which may cause a slide in centric. This, too, is important from an orthodontic viewpoint.

The mucosae of the lips, cheeks and palate are inspected with special attention for white patches, ulcerations or discolorations. The tongue is examined for size, shape, patches or ulcers and the patient is asked to protrude the tongue and attention is paid to any deviation to one side and, if this is so, the cause is ascertained. The gingivae are examined: colour, form and texture are important. Crevices (or pockets) should be gently explored using a blunt probe, and especially useful are periodontal probes (of the Williams type) marked in millimetres. This should be introduced into the crevice or pocket with the probe tip and blade parallel to the long axis of the tooth. Another useful probe is the Svenska which has a measuring scale with which it is possible to read the pocket depths directly. (*Fig. 6.*)

It is doubtful whether there is ever any need to use a sharp explorer or probe. One's own early recollections of being instructed on examining for caries was being told to use a needle sharp probe which was 'leaned on' pretty heavily, and if it stuck then this was a 'cavity' requiring filling. The question of what constitutes a cavity or indeed caries attack is one which must exercise all the judgement of anyone wishing to practise preventive dentistry. Is the sticky fissure merely a deep enamel-lined cleft, or is there a breach of surface with loss of enamel, and dentine under attack? If this is taking place in the depth of a fissure, how does one know? If one uses a sharp probe to get down to the bottom of a fissure might it not break through the enamel at the base? What is going to be the consequence of leaving it all alone? It is difficult to make out any argument for the sharp pointed probe.

However, so-called 'sticky' areas should be noted on the patient's chart with the date of observation and they should be checked periodically for extension, or invasion of tooth substance.

A similar need for care is necessary when probing for pocket depth. According to Prichard (1979) it often happens that the probe goes through the junctional epithelium into the connective tissue. Also when contemplating our treatment plan we should consider that pockets and bony defects are the result of disease, but are not the active disease process. Schroeder and Listgarten (1977) state 'Periodontal probing may be valuable in assessing the periodontal status of a patient, (but) the measurements obtained do not bear any relationship to actual pocket depth and only infrequently correspond to the most coronal level of the connective tissue attachment. While in a clinically normal state the level is markedly underestimated because the probe only penetrates part of the width of the junctional epithelium, in cases of overt periodontitis this level is overestimated to a variable degree.' The import of all this is that all our probing should be performed gently with a blunt or round ended probe and the minimum of pressure. However, it must be emphasized that more harm is done to patients by *not* probing and therefore missing frank periodontal disease.

DIAGNOSIS AND TREATMENT PLANNING

4. *Radiography*

Other diagnostic aids should be used. It may be said that every new patient requires complete full mouth radiography of approximately 14 films. Panoramic radiography enables a preliminary examination with prognosis to be carried out very rapidly (*Fig.* 7). This is not only valuable in the saving of time but total radiation is reduced, and of course it is very simple for the patient (especially children) as no films are placed in the mouth. An ideal initial radiographic examination today is one panoramic film and two bitewings. This gives an 80 per cent reduction on the radiation effect of a 14 film full mouth study. In the standard intra-oral film examination the use of long cone techniques as much as possible will give more accurate images (*Fig.* 8). The use of bitewing films with built in or with adhesive bite tabs combined with long cone on the tube gives a simple method of achieving coverage of many posterior teeth with accurate technique. An excellent and accurate bitewing film holder is the lightweight plastic Kwikbite (Hawe Dental). The use of XCP bitewing and other holders (which many patients dislike) is not necessary in this method.

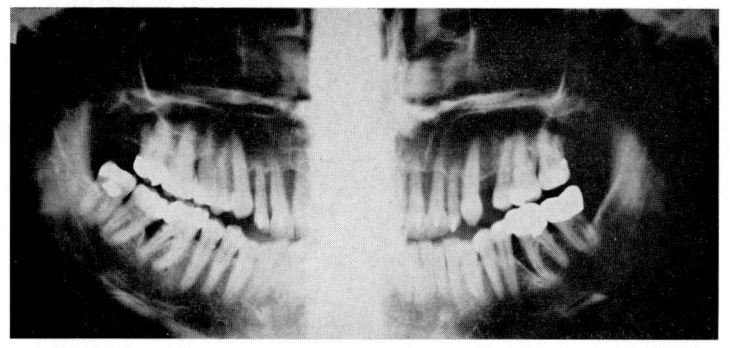

Fig. 7. A panoramic survey gives a considerable amount of information quickly and with low radiation dosage. Note the clear indication of the alveolar level.

At this stage the dentist should have a good idea what the patient's 'needs' are from the point of view of bringing the state of the mouth as close as possible to the ideals established by his professional training. It would be surprising if the patient's 'wants' coincided with the dentist's ideas of his 'needs'.

At the preliminary planning discussion there will be a further establishment of communication, and the dentist should explain to the patient the need for an initial course of training in a preventive approach combined with the health preparation of the mouth by himself or the hygienist. There is strong argument in favour of the

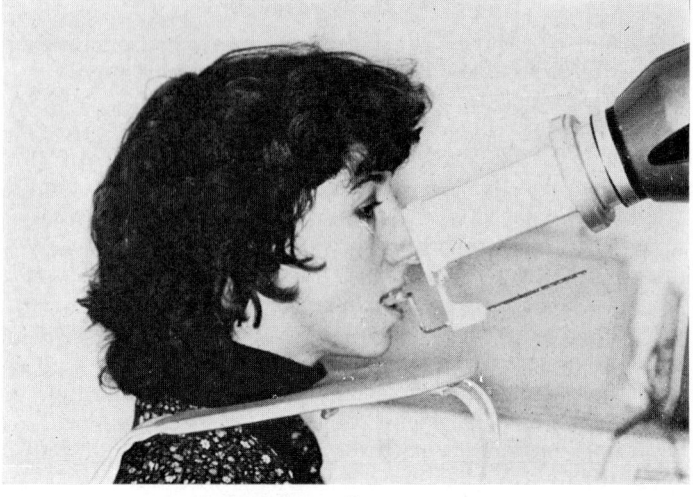

PREVENTIVE DENTISTRY

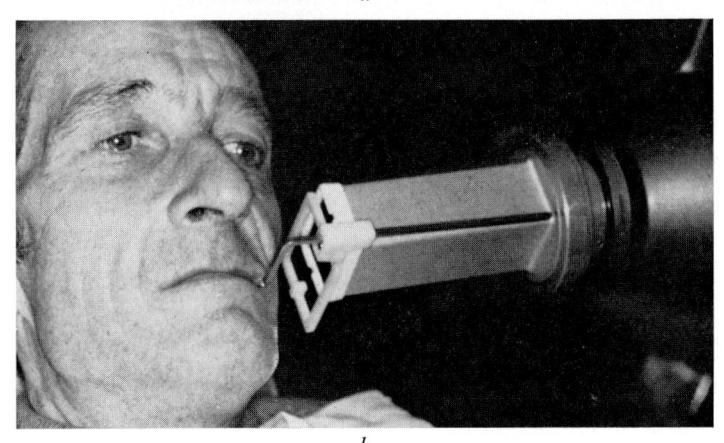

Fig. 8. *a*, Long cone aligned for upper incisor radiograph. Reduced area of radiation. Note the lead platform shield under the chin protecting the rest of the body from stray radiation. *b*, 'Cone' aligned with Rinn holder for posterior teeth.

early preparation of the mouth (i.e. scaling, plaque control, training in home care) being carried out by someone other than the dentist who will be concerned in any reconstruction techniques. In this way the important nature of the initial procedures is emphasized and also there is no temptation or pressure on the dentist to start his definitive restorations too early with often disastrous results. Indeed, in the obviously neglected cases with poor care and recurrent caries, or existing periodontal disease, the patient is told that treatment, other than emergency or temporary, may not begin until there is a satisfactory outcome to this first stage.

Cheney (1977) describes the necessary changes from the traditional approach where little emphasis was placed on the role of the patient except as a passive receptor of treatment to one in which account is taken of the personality and behaviour patterns of both patient and dentist with a treatment plan varied to fit individual needs. He outlines these changes as follows:

1. *Traditional model: Clinical treatment by dentist*

	Doctor	Patient (behaviour/personality)	Treatment Plan
Change factors:	None	None	Same for all patients

2. *Attempt to change the behaviour or motivate the patient towards a 'new' way of dental care.* (This is typical of the methods used in the recent initial preventive dentistry wave)

	Doctor	Patient	Treatment Plan
Change factors:	None	Maximal	Same for all patients

3. *Recommended current approach* puts maximum emphasis on knowing each patient, analysing personalities and then tailoring the final treatment plan

	Doctor	Patient	Treatment Plan
Change factors:	None	None	Modified for each patient

At reassessment following a preliminary programme there may be considerable modifications made to any previous tentative plan. This will be based on the patient's demonstrated ability to cope with the care of the potentially restored mouth. If not, the type of treatment should be tailored to the ability and the interest which has been shown.

Also, as Young (1965) has stated: 'If the (dentist's) objectives are too far above the expectations of the patient, treatment may be rejected entirely or fail if accepted. A prescribed course of periodontal therapy may be the "ideal" technical treatment for a patient with advanced periodontal disease . . . yet be unrealistic and unwise without proper motivation. In this instance, the alternative of extractions and complete dentures may well be "ideal" from the standpoint of optimum oral health to a specific human being.'

The dentist must also be conscious of another factor, that of his own technical ability to carry out any planned treatment. He should otherwise consider referral of the patient to someone he considers to be more capable of carrying out a particular procedure. He may of course opt for a treatment plan which involves simpler procedures, meanwhile informing the patient of the more elaborate plan if this is appropriate to the patient's case.

Thus, in summary, we may say that a possible successful treatment plan will involve a compromise between the patient's 'wants', the patient's 'needs', the treatment possibilities assessed on the results of reviewing the patient's attitude to home care and initial preparation of the mouth, and the dentist's technical capabilities.

Any omission of consideration of these factors will 'neglect to provide beforehand against the occurrence of failure and the re-establishment of disease'.

REFERENCES

Binnie W. H. (1976) A perspective of oral cancer. *Proc. Roy. Soc. Med.* **69,** 737–740.

Binnie W. H., Cawson R. A., Hill G. B. and Soaper A. E. (1972) *Oral Cancer in England and Wales.* Studies on Medical and Population Subjects No. 23. London, H.M.S.O.

Cheney H. G. (1977) Effect of patient behaviour and personality on treatment planning. *Dent. Clin. North Am.* **21,** 531–538.

Prichard John F. (1979) *The Diagnosis and Treatment of Periodontal Disease.* Philadelphia, Saunders. p. 99.

Schroeder H. E. and Listgarten M. A. (1977) *Fine Structure of the Developing Epithelial Attachment of Human Teeth,* 2nd Ed. Basel, Karger. p. 111.

Silverston J. F. and Burgell F. G. (1976) Probing of pockets related to the attachment level. *J. Periodont.* **74,** 281.

Young W. (1965) Motivating patients to accept preventive services. *Dent. Clin. North Am.* **9,** 523–533.

CHAPTER 3

DENTAL PLAQUE AND ITS CONTROL

IT is now generally recognized that dental plaque is involved in the pathogenicity of both caries and periodontal disease. The exact mechanism of periodontal disease progression in relation to plaque is the subject of much research work. There seems to be agreement among researchers that periodontal disease is associated with the presence of bacterial colonies on the surfaces above and in the gingival crevice initiating an inflammatory reaction due to the toxic products of organisms in the plaque; the action of endotoxins and host reactions to the antigens.

The still widely held view in respect of caries initiation is the action by micro-organisms in the plaque which is in intimate relationship with the tooth surface. These organisms act on sucrose products entering the plaque after carbohydrate ingestion, and form acids which at the critical pH level (below 5·5) bring about enamel dissolution. Our preventive efforts relative to caries involve increasing the acid solubility resistance of the tooth surface (by the use of fluorides), carbohydrate limitation, and plaque reduction, but when we consider our methods of prevention in relation to periodontal disease we find that we have as yet one measure only which has universal practical application—plaque removal.

Plaque formation does not take place haphazardly but in a reasonably orderly manner. A pellicle derived from the saliva or gingival fluid first forms on the teeth. This pellicle is a thin, clear cuticle and is composed mainly of glycoproteins. Very soon after its formation, bacteria of the coccus type (streptococci largely) are attracted to the pellicle which has a 'sticky' surface, i.e. one which enables colonies of organisms to be anchored. These organisms divide and form colonies. Attachment of the micro-organisms is further enhanced by the production by the bacteria of dextrans as by-products of metabolic activity. Later other types of organisms are attracted to the mass and a dense mixed flora, now also containing filamentous forms, results.

Plaque may attach to the teeth supragingivally, or subgingivally in the gingival crevice, or in periodontal pockets. Both types of plaque may vary because of the differing intake of substances from the saliva and diet in supragingival plaque, and from gingival exudate, etc. in the subgingival area.

The early form of plaque is said to be more cariogenic while the later form may be concerned in the initiation of periodontal disease.

It has been known for a long time that periodontal disease is largely preventable, and that in the early stages treatment can be very simple. With further progression of the disease, that is with increased destruction of the supporting tissues, there is need for more involved therapy, but until quite a late stage success can be achieved in arresting the disease and retaining the teeth in good function. Periodontal care, however, is dependent for its continued success on awareness, diligence and constant reappraisal by the dentist and the patient.

We have reached a stage in caries control where it is possible to reduce substantially the caries attack and with some goodwill on all sides it is possible to visualize a not-too-distant time when dental decay is no longer the enormous problem that it has been to this day. And all this can seemingly be achieved with very little active co-operation on the part of the patient. If we are to control or treat periodontal disease however, very considerable help is required from the patient and without it treatment is nearly always likely to fail.

For many years dentists were taught the importance of thorough calculus and debris removal and its beneficial effects on the health of the gingiva. During one's own training the term 'dental plaque' had not come into use, but very good results were obtained with debris and calculus removal all those years ago, and long before. But a number of cases responded either very slowly or not at all. The therapy for these patients, as well as the very advanced cases where by rule of thumb any pocket of over 3 mm in depth was not considered treatable conservatively, was to carry out a gingivectomy procedure. Unfortunately, many of these cases relapsed post-surgically and one of the reasons for this (but not the only reason) was that the basic cause—bacteria—had not been evaluated and eliminated. The dentist and periodontist were not aware that bacterial plaque was frequently invisible and so they were too easily satisfied that oral hygiene procedures were being assiduously carried out. Therefore, the failures were often considered to be due to systemic factors and there followed a period of intense activity in which various hormones, male, female and other imagined deficiencies, were either applied topically or given parenterally.

Much research has been carried out, and continues, into the obviously potentially rewarding line of plaque prevention (by antibiotics and chemical methods)—e.g. the experimental use of chlorhexidine—but as yet there is no acceptable material available for routine use. Thus there is no periodontal equivalent at present to the use of fluoride compounds in various forms in caries prevention. The importance of this latter measure is that it offers the health services—at the practice, community and public health levels —opportunity for controlling disease to a large extent without putting responsibility on the patient. This we cannot achieve in relation to periodontal disease.

There is a vast difference between results of research using animals and subsequent application in humans. We can all remember the excitement aroused by dextranase, which was going to prevent plaque formation and hence subsequent plaque-mediated diseases. Many of us had requests from the public for dextranase *now*, coupled with complaints that we were 'behind the times' because it was not part of our armamentarium. Fortunately, long-term experience has taught the value of waiting for reasonable assessment of newspaper 'miracle treatments'. Most recent work has regrettably shown a lack of success with dextranase even as a plaque inhibitor.

Well documented and acceptable research studies, which have been amply confirmed (and in fact were a matter of general observation by most dentists), were carried out by Löe and Schiott (1970). They demonstrated that by keeping the teeth completely free from plaque inflammation of the gingivae could be prevented. Conversely, by ordering a cessation of tooth cleaning in their subjects, plaque was allowed to accumulate in the gingival crevice regions and gingivitis ensued.

Löe and others also demonstrated that if brushing was so effectively carried out that all plaque was removed, then recolonization did not take place appreciably until 48 hours had elapsed and therefore, in this instance, it was acceptable to brush every other day. As, however, this degree of cleanliness is an almost impossible attainment with nearly all our patients, one should concentrate on training them to a standard of plaque removal which is effective enough to allow once-a-day brushing.

Much of this and other work on plaque reverses some of our own previously held views. We have all for years told our patients to brush after meals, especially after taking sugary substances. However, if there were no plaque on the teeth before consuming the meal, there would be no matrix to hold the sugars and other substances in contact with the teeth. Thus if we could achieve effective complete plaque elimination by brushing and other accessory means, there is a strong argument for this being carried out *before* meals. But until we do achieve a satisfactory plaque control score, it is probably better to stick to the conventional method and ask the patient to remove not only plaque but also the potentially harmful sugar residue after meals.

Axelsson and Lindhe (1974) (1978) conducted classic investigations where in one study children, and in the other adults, were instructed in daily home mouth care supported by frequent visits for professional cleaning by a trained auxiliary with local applications of fluoride. Motivation was reinforced and repeated training

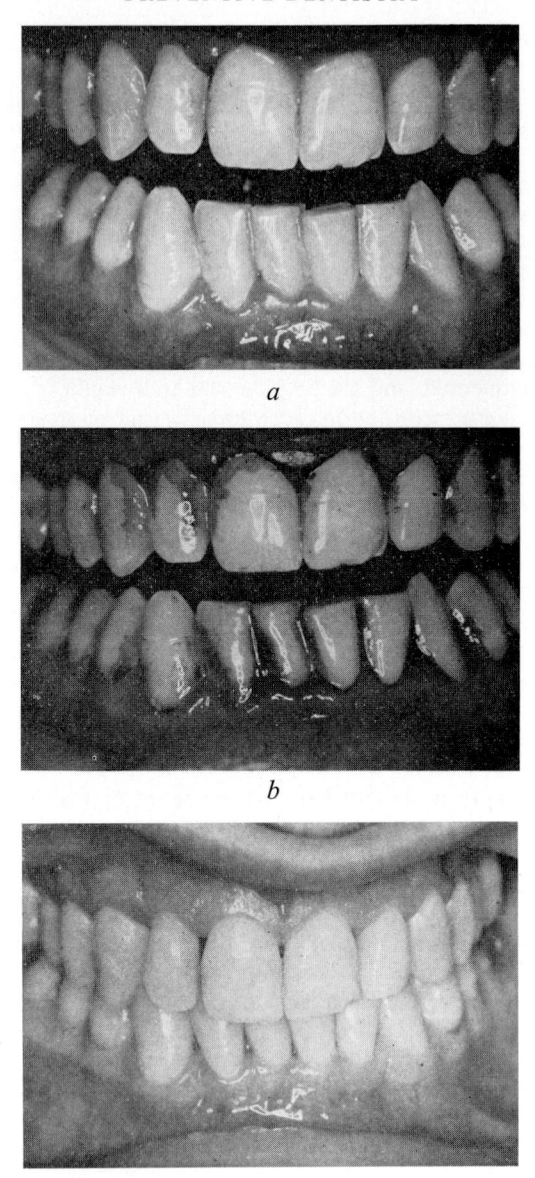

Fig. 9. *a*, The gingivae are inflamed and bleeding in a teenage patient. *b*, The bacterial film and deposits are disclosed using Talbot's iodine, which is very dramatic. *c*, The improvement brought about by careful brushing after repeated oral hygiene training.

in oral hygiene procedures was given. The results were dramatic reduction in caries and gingival inflammation. These results show the importance of repeated visits for professional plaque removal and reinforcement. It confirms the findings that most of us have noticed clinically that frequent and short-interval recall is of considerable help in maintaining oral health even in those with poor co-operation in home care.

DISCLOSING PLAQUE

Most patients are unaware of the bacterial film on the teeth and equate 'dirt' with discolorations of varying degrees. The dentist, too, is often not aware that apparently clean-looking teeth have heavy deposits. It is essential to make these deposits visible:

1. To confirm to the patient the presence of a harmful film and hence facilitate instruction on its removal.
2. To enable the dentist or hygienist, during scaling and polishing procedures, to confirm that the tooth surfaces are free from all deposits.

It was the simple expedient of disclosing media which changed the direction of periodontal care, and hence we owe a debt to Dr. Sumter Arnim (1963) for this introduction (*Figs.* 9, 10). Unfortunately, the patient was almost immediately burdened with the total responsibility of plaque removal, and thus the patient's workload doubled or trebled. But the results were very good indeed. It became possible to treat many cases of gingivitis at the bleeding

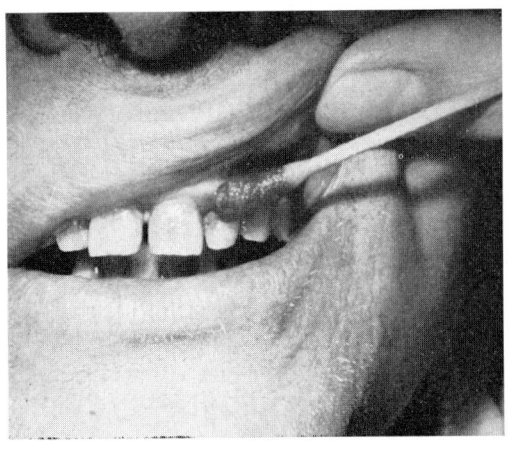

Fig. 10. Disclosing solution is more acceptable than tablets. It may be applied with a cotton tip.

stage often with nothing more than very careful training in the effective use of the toothbrush. We know, therefore, that the patient has a fundamental role to play in plaque removal, both in treatment and maintenance of the restored tissues. It is not sufficient, however, merely to tell the patient to carry out these procedures. When a patient has been accepted for treatment the dentist has a basic and never-ending responsibility in motivating and encouraging the patient's role in that dental care and this applies to all forms of dental treatment.

The desirable properties of a disclosing substance should be:
- *a.* Ability to stain plaque selectively so that this will stand out from the cleaner portions of the teeth and surroundings.
- *b.* Absence of prolonged retained staining of the rest of the oral structures—lips, cheeks, tongue.
- *c.* Anterior tooth coloured fillings should not be adversely affected.
- *d.* Taste must be acceptable.
- *e.* No harmful effects on the mucous membrane, nor should there be a possibility of harm caused by accidental swallowing of the substance or from possible allergic reaction.

Some Disclosing Agents

Pink Disclosing Tablets

Dr. Sumter Arnim introduced what are termed in the U.S.A. 'disclosing wafers', which are in effect 'tablets' of erythrocin food dye—an acceptable food additive officially termed 'F.D.C. Red No. 3' (a 6 per cent solution in water).

Iodine Based Solutions

A formula is given in Appendix 1. The advantage of the iodine based solutions is that their effect is very dramatic. Plaque is stained deeply—brown or black—and the associated inflamed gingivae also show up as dark areas. It is then very easy to demonstrate the ill-effects of the plaque. The discoloration in fact disappears in a few minutes. This type of disclosing agent is excellent for clinical photography.

Another important advantage (hence lack of pressure selling by supply houses) is low cost. It can be made up by the local pharmacist. Two possible disadvantages are:
1. Some patients are allergic to iodine based products, and
2. Some find the taste objectionable.

Other Commercial Disclosing Agents

After much experience of disclosing agents, the prescription or issue of disclosing *tablets* for chewing or sucking was abandoned many years ago. The indiscriminate staining of lips, cheek and tongue, which lasted for hours, was disliked by patients and they quickly discontinued the use of their tablets, often while still professing to be employing them. Similar objections apply to solutions for rinsing. Hence all acceptable disclosing agents are those which can be applied just to the areas to be checked—usually by a cotton tip.

The dentist should be able to evaluate all these new products by trying out samples (on himself—this will also help his own plaque control!). A most effective solution would appear to be Displaque (*Fig.* 11). It selectively stains varying thicknesses of plaque in different colours. Kieser and Wade (1976) state that, 'there are readily available cheap food colourants which are quite as effective in disclosing plaque as the best of the proprietary agents and difficulty in obtaining the latter should not, therefore, be a handicap to the implementation of improved oral hygiene practices.'

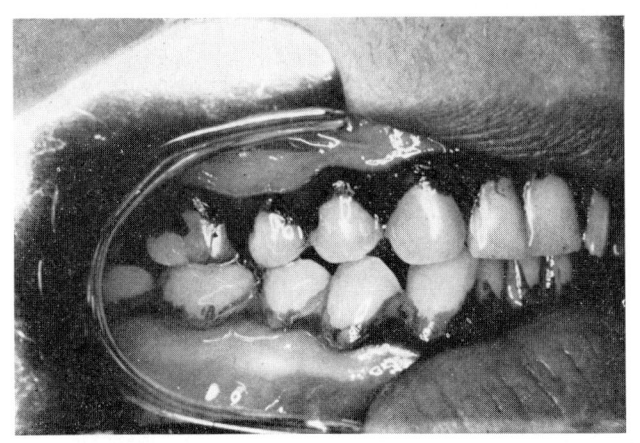

Fig. 11. Differential staining showing various thicknesses and maturity of plaque (Displaque).

THE PLAKLITE (*Fig.* 12): This apparatus consists of a small mains operated lamp which gives a white light through a special dichroic filter. A bottle of a fluorescein based solution is supplied and two drops of this are introduced into the mouth and the patient is instructed to swish it in the saliva all around the mouth. The indicator fluid has a special affinity for plaque but is relatively invisible until the light makes it appear with a greenish yellow glow. The effect is startling and dramatic and may well be responsible for an added keenness to remove the offending glow.

It is useful, but not always necessary, to record the patient's plaque score or index. Comparison of such scores at intervals

PREVENTIVE DENTISTRY

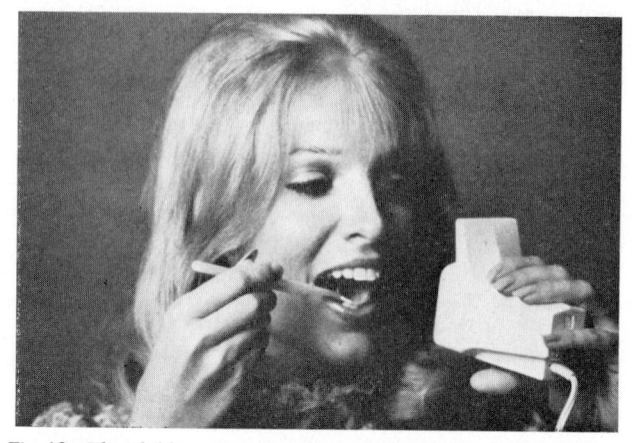

Fig. 12. *The Plaklite.* A mains connected lamp used with a fluorescein based solution. Two drops of fluorescein are swished around the teeth. The plaque absorbs the fluorescein and glows when the special light from the Plaklite is concentrated on it.

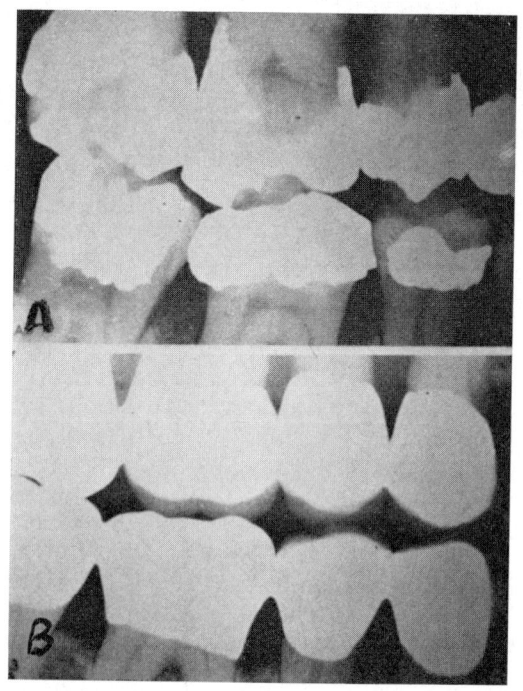

Fig. 13. *a,* Poor filling margins responsible for periodontal breakdown. *b,* Acceptable margins and embrasures.

during treatment will indicate the progress made in oral hygiene training. That of Silness and Loe (1964) is often used.

0 = no plaque.
1 = a film of plaque at gingival level detectable by scraping with a probe or by the use of a disclosing agent.
2 = moderate accumulation of deposits within the pockets or on the margins which can readily be seen.
3 = heavy accumulation of soft material filling the niche between the tooth surface and the gingival margin or fills the interdental area.

The index is recorded for all surfaces of the selected teeth—mesial, distal and oral and vestibular. The scores for all the surfaces of the selected teeth are totalled and divided by the number of teeth to arrive at the Plaque Index.

The gingival index of Loe and Silness (1963) corresponds very closely to the plaque index and scores from 0 for normal gingivae, to 3 for severe inflammation and ulceration.

MINIMIZING PLAQUE FORMATION

Having demonstrated the presence of plaque the dentist's responsibility is one of (*a*) removing it, (*b*) ensuring that the patient can remove it and prevent its formation, and (*c*) so to order the anatomy of the mouth and teeth, where possible, to discourage bacterial growth and retention. Attention should therefore be paid to the following factors which favour plaque retention:

1. Filling overhangs (*Fig.* 13).
2. Open or poor contacts between teeth.
3. Unfavourable crown contours.
4. Cavities in teeth.
5. Gingival craters following destructive gingival disease.
6. High fraenum insertions interfering with brush placement.
7. Malaligned teeth making some areas difficult to reach (*Fig.* 14).
8. Ill-fitting dentures, orthodontic and other appliances which are neglected (*Fig.* 15).
9. Incomplete lip closure (*Fig.* 32, p. 76).
10. Excessive sucrose intake.

The greatest trouble should be taken to facilitate and encourage effective toothbrushing which is our main method of attacking the plaque problem. This will be dealt with very fully in the following sections. All the disclosants discussed are a means to encourage effective brushing, and thus without the latter all disclosants would be a waste of time and money.

There is no doubt that many people have a well developed oral self-cleansing ability, i.e. the removal of debris by tongue and salivary activity without the use of accessory aids. They have a fine oral awareness and will be worried by the presence of a small amount of food or other material on or between the teeth. Such subjects, if a partial denture (however well made) is fitted, will complain for a week or two about food collecting around the appliance and the necessity of cleaning it carefully after each meal. But they will, in a very short time, no longer complain and examination reveals that they have developed the ability to clean around the denture with the tongue. This is so frequent that it has become an integral part of the initial advice and reassurance to the patient on the first insertion of a new partial denture.

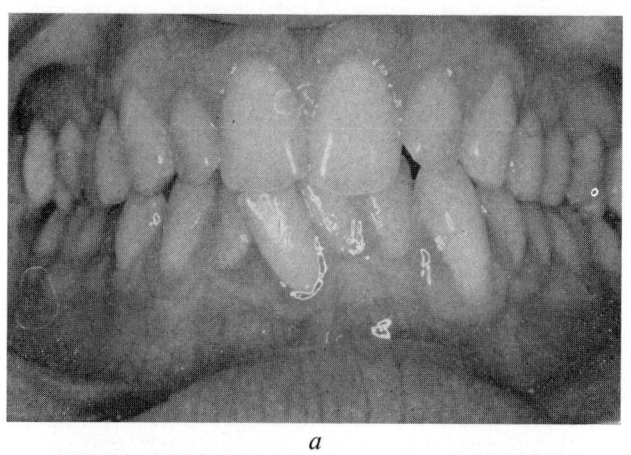

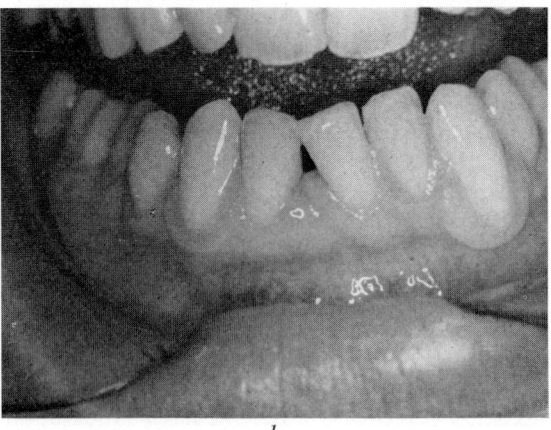

Fig. 14. Toothbrushing rendered more effective by the judicious removal of an interfering tooth. *b*, Note the improvement in gingival condition.

Conversely, there are those with diminished oral perception, and some with almost none. These have no sense of what is going on in their mouths. Some will present with lost molar crowns, fractured teeth with sharp edges and yet will have no concept of anything wrong. The two illustrations (*Fig.* 16) are those of physicians, one male (*Fig.* 16*a*) the other female (*Fig.* 16*b*) who have no idea of how bad their mouths were! The female was quite good-looking and only 26 years of age. She wore a partial upper denture with clasps and occlusal rests. On a number of occasions when her mouth was examined it was found that the denture was only partly inserted and the clasps and rests must have been projecting beyond the teeth and presented a hazard to tongue and cheeks. On no occasion was the patient aware that the denture was not in place. She was unaware that one of the septic root apices was visible through a large defect in the alveolus (arrowed in *Fig.* 16*b*). Such an extreme case can be an impossible subject for oral hygiene training and thus frequent attendance for professional care is essential. Some intermediate types can be made aware of their oral state, but with difficulty. We have found few methods by which we can create 'oral awareness' with certainty in such cases.

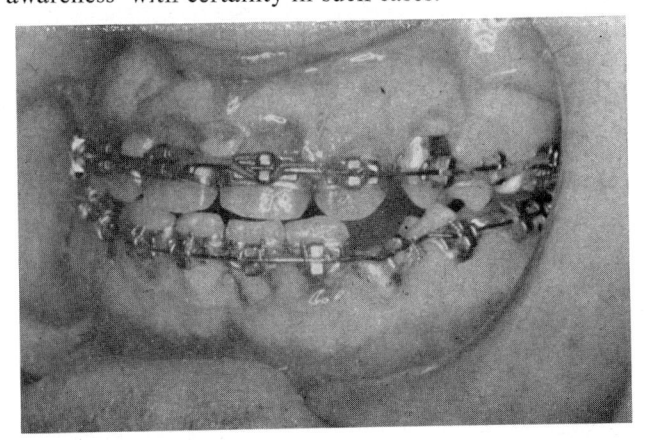

Fig. 15. Extra care is necessary when fixed orthodontic appliances are used. In this case insufficient emphasis was given to oral hygiene procedures.

METHODS OF PLAQUE CONTROL
1. Chemical.
2. Irrigation.
3. Mechanical.

1. *Chemical*

Although many antibiotics, used topically, can reduce plaque incidence quite considerably, the dangers of developing resistant strains of organisms, sensitization and candidiasis, render the use of such medication open to serious objection. Chlorhexidine in a concentration of 0·2 per cent used daily as a mouth rinse has been shown to be effective in preventing plaque formation in patients where other oral hygiene measures had been discontinued. However the side effects such as discoloration of teeth and some restorations, and the undesirable taste limits the general adoption at present of such a rinse.

Current commercial products of this nature, in order to minimize

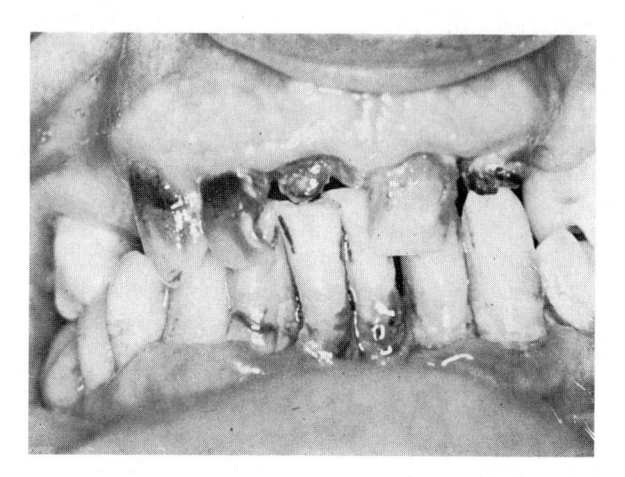

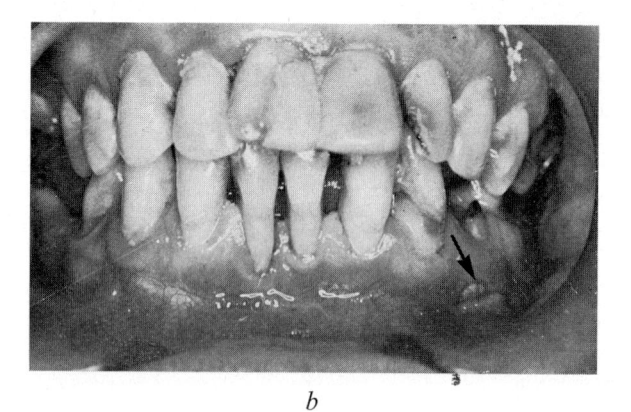

Fig. 16. *a*, *b*, The teeth of physicians (*see text*). In *b* arrow points to sinus in patient's lower left premolar region.

the above problems, have diluted the active ingredient to the point of reduced efficacy. However research along these lines must eventually bear fruit and offers great hope.

2. Water Irrigation
(*Fig.* 17)

The use of water irrigation appliances, which are expensive, has very little justification in oral hygiene training. There is no question that they do not remove plaque and, although some of the manufacturers

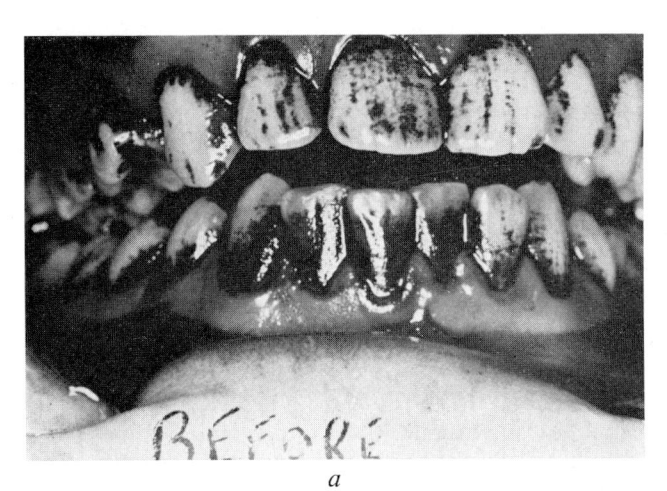

Fig. 17. *a*, Plaque stained with Talbot's iodine before using pulsating water irrigation outfit (Water Pik). *b*, Plaque remaining after prolonged use of the outfits.

have modified their claims to that of apparently changing the character of the plaque (difficult to check), the trouble involved would not appear to warrant yet another chore for the patient. There is no doubt that these devices have led both dentists and patients to become complacent about leaving deep pockets because 'pressure sprays will clean them out'. Regrettably this belief has often led to neglect of definitive treatment and occasionally acute abscess formation. It may be of interest to note that the Water Pik is no longer on the American Dental Association 'accepted list'. (Council on Dental Materials and Devices, 1974.)

Schmid (1980) says 'water irrigators are not capable of removing any appreciable amounts of stainable plaque from tooth surfaces and, therefore should not be recommended for prevention of caries, gingivitis, periodontitis'.

It would take too long to give lists of all the gadgets and devices available. Some are described in Appendix 1. The dentist is advised to be wary and to give a prolonged trial to such appliances and materials, however highly recommended by salesmen. If everyone is still happy after one month he can possibly consider its further use.

3. *Mechanical Methods*

Polishing—a Fundamental Necessity

One of the most important aspects of prevention is the provision of smooth well-polished surfaces which become plaque coated and stained less easily than rough or unpolished surfaces. This cannot be over-emphasized, and yet this is dealt with only rarely in publications.

One uses polishing techniques in the following situations:

1. Natural tooth surfaces.
2. The filled tooth, i.e. finishing the restoration.
3. Artificial dentures.

Some basic principles should be observed.

It is almost always necessary to use techniques and materials which avoid the production of heat. Both tooth substance and restorative materials will be adversely affected by overheating. Therefore, where possible slow speeds should be used and composition of rubber wheels, pastes, etc., should be checked to confirm that there are no ingredients which may be harmful to tooth surface or to filling materials (e.g. amalgams may be seriously affected by sulphur, which is contained in some rubber polishing discs).

Harsh polishing pastes such as pumice should not, in normal circumstances, be used on enamel surfaces, unless the severe scratching which results may be somewhat desirable as in etching techniques used in the currently developing methods of incisal tip rebuilding with composite materials, or in fissure sealing.

Polishing Methods

Armamentarium

Polishing instruments and materials.
Disclosing solutions.
For a list of the above *see* Appendix 1.

1. *Natural Tooth Surfaces*

Since well polished smooth enamel surfaces retain plaque less well than rough surfaces, it is necessary to polish all tooth surfaces after the removal of plaque and calculus which has been carried out as a routine prophylaxis or as part of a periodontal treatment. Many of the commercially available prophylaxis and polishing pastes are too abrasive, even flour of pumice, and will remove the more acid resistant surface layer or scratch it (Massler, 1969). It has been shown that more enamel abrasion may result from dentists' polishing than from toothbrush and dentifrice usage (Brasch et al., 1969). This would support those patients who complained that 'my teeth seem to get dirtier much quicker since I had them cleaned by the dentist'. It is also some sort of basis for another belief that scaling and polishing 'takes the enamel off'. Of course, all these complaints were, and still are, hotly denied as 'old wives' tales', but occasionally there is an element of truth, perhaps wrongly interpreted, in these beliefs.

The investigation above confirmed our own feelings which had led to the abandonment many years ago of the use of conventional pumice-containing polishing pastes. Additionally, motor driven polishing brushes are rarely used on enamel, the finishing polish being carried out with small webbed cups (of the Crescent type) held in a special angle polishing head or an old contra-angle handpiece kept specially for this purpose.

Therefore, 'safe' polishing materials such as zirconium silicate (e.g. Zircate), tin oxide or even zinc oxide should be used. In the case of a scaling procedure which is prolonged over three or four visits and where, say, a quadrant is completed at each visit, neglect of polishing at the termination of each visit will allow plaque to accumulate as readily as before. In addition, the feel of well-polished teeth gives the patient a greater incentive to carry out home care procedures in order to keep the present smooth clean feeling for as long as possible.

The procedure for polishing the teeth therefore follows the pattern:

a. Very careful scaling, and if an ultrasonic unit is used much stain may be removed by judicious use of the tip. It should be remembered that deeply pitted stains are unlikely to be removed by a mechanical polishing method such as the motor driven brush and paste without reducing the surface of the surrounding enamel markedly.

b. Where possible, the proximal surfaces of the teeth gingival to the contact points are polished with strips. Anterior teeth are much easier to strip polish in this way and a medium width (4 mm) 'Zirc' hygienists finishing strip, centre gapped, is very effective and easy to use. These strips may be passed through the embrasure under the contact point and if necessary a narrow strip (2·5 mm) may be used. In order to save time all the left proximal surfaces may be polished with the same strip which may be brought back and reversed to polish all the right proximal surfaces.

c. A disclosing solution is then applied to the teeth to be polished and the patient asked to rinse this away after a few seconds. Any obvious gross stains may be removed by hand instrumentation. The teeth are then polished by using a rubber cup loaded with zirconium silicate paste (or powder, made up to a paste with water) running at fairly low speed. All surfaces are polished and the edges of the cup introduced into the embrasures to polish the proximal surfaces as well as possible. The occlusal surfaces should not be forgotten.

d. A final polish (e.g. at termination of treatment in the adult) should include the use of a fluoride-containing polishing paste which can be made up by adding two drops of a freshly mixed 10 per cent solution of stannous fluoride to Zircate prophylaxis paste in a dappen glass, or failing the availability of stannous fluoride, commercial APF solution can be used. A disclosing solution is again used and any residual stains are repolished. The patient is asked to see the result after using a disclosing solution on clean teeth and then to run his tongue over the surfaces. 'This is your target from now on', he is told. (*Fig.* 18.)

2. *Finishing and Polishing the Restoration*

Only cast gold restorations have the edge strength to cover enamel margins in thin layers without the risk of the restoration margins fracturing and leaving either the tooth-filling junction exposed or, worse, bare enamel rods. Thus restorations of the more brittle materials, amalgams, silicates, composites, should be inserted in cavities in which no enamel bevel has been prepared, in order to avoid the risk of bare enamel rods without their 30 microns or so of acid resistant enamel surface being attacked by recurrent caries.

Amalgam

It used to be considered undesirable to burnish the surface and margins of freshly inserted amalgam because this was said to weaken the margins. Recent work has indicated that burnishing may be acceptable as it has been shown that it decreased the mercury content and the porosity at the margins (Kanai, 1966). The better the carving and finishing at the insertion stage the less grinding and trimming (with the risk of overheating) at the later polishing stage.

Therefore the occlusal surface should be carved (some dentists use

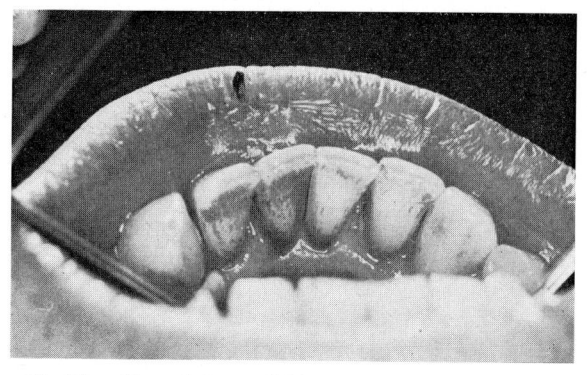

Fig. 18. The effect of fine polishing of enamel. The incisors on the right of the picture have been polished with zirconium silicate paste, while those on the left of the picture have been polished with pumice type pastes. Three weeks later the photograph shows less staining on the zirconium silicate side.

a sharp scalpel), and burnished if desired. The surface is then wiped with a dry cotton bud to remove any free mercury.

If the amalgam filling involves the proximal (mesial or distal) surface this should be dealt with first. After removal of the matrix band and wedge, the proximal gingival margins are stroked with the side of a curved probe from buccal and lingual aspects to remove any excess filling or slight irregularities. Following this, a narrow (2·5 mm) extra-fine grit polishing strip is passed through the embrasure under the contact point (and if this cannot be passed there is going to be an 'embrasure problem' as described in the chapter on preventive aspects of restorative dentistry) and the strip is pulled buccolingually along the gingival margin to smooth this off while the amalgam is still reasonably soft. In this way one of the commonest dentist-associated causes of localized periodontal breakdown—the filling overhang—is avoided. Care must be taken, of course, not to interfere with the form of the contact areas between the teeth, provided that they are satisfactory.

Finishing and polishing is carried out after 48 hours and the surface is smoothed with finishing burs or stones run slowly in the handpiece. Fine cuttle or sandpaper discs may be used, run wet if possible, followed by special amalgam polishing cones (Dedeco).

The filling should then be polished (together with the contiguous enamel surface) with mildly abrasive pastes and preferably there should be a final polish of the restored surface, especially the margins, with a fluoride containing paste and this may effect replacement of any fluoride which may have been removed during the filling procedure (Horowitz and Lucye, 1966).

Gold Inlays

Usually these will have been polished in the laboratory and should require no finishing or polishing in the mouth. All margins should be carefully burnished, however, and if possible the inlay should be cemented with a fluoride-containing cement, e.g. Fluorothin (S.S.W.) or Poly F (De Trey). At the following visit the margins should be gently polished with a zirconium silicate plus fluoride paste in a rubber cup (*see also* p. 114).

Anterior Fillings

Whether these are composite, silicate or direct acrylic fillings, the main hazard is the same. Any overhangs at or below the gingival margin may be undetectable and these have been a frequent cause of localized gingival inflammation. It is therefore important to wedge the proximal areas very carefully after insertion of the material and subsequently to seek out any excess with a probe. A very fine diamond tip should be reserved for the purpose of clearing this excess. Messing and Ray (1972) recommended the use of sharp scalpels to shape off the excess composite. But the newer, much harder composite materials, some of them light activated, e.g. Visio Dispers, are not easily trimmed, even with diamond instruments and therefore margins should be carefully wedged or, in the case of light polymerized materials, smoothed off before application of the lamp. Fine polishing of composite fillings is difficult. The main surface is best left undisturbed with 'cellulose acetate strip finish'. Should this not be possible, smooth carbide stones are followed by 3M composite finishing discs—first the medium grit, followed by the fine. A fine rubber polishing wheel is also marketed for finishing these fillings.

3. *Removable Dentures*

The polishing of dentures is, of course, less immediately fraught with danger to other structures because this is carried out in the dental laboratory. The following is a summary of the more important aspects of denture polishing as it relates to tissue care:

a. The non-fitting surface should be polished to a very high gloss, and in the case of acrylic dentures care must be taken at all times in order not to overheat the material.

b. The fitting surface of acrylic dentures should have all the roughness and indentations removed and the surface should be polished to a reasonable smoothness. There should be no 'pimples' or excrescences in the surface as these will irritate the mucosa during the slight movement all dentures make under stress. Neither should there be any acute depressions which may collect plaque or other accumulation or organisms.

c. All sharp points including the dreaded 'collets' should be removed. These points variously can damage tongue, cheek and the gingiva relating to the region of the pointed denture base of clasps. The inside of clasps should be highly polished and the patient should have a separate careful demonstration of clasp polishing as part of home care routine.

Fixed Bridgework

This should of course be polished before final insertion. Any subsequent polishing would require the same attention as that noted for inlays.

It is therefore to be hoped that there has been adequate demonstration here that careful polishing is not just an extra that may or may not be thrown in 'if there is time', but is an important part of all our restorative and preventive procedures.

THE TOOTHBRUSH AND ITS USE

There is a multitude of different shapes, textures, sizes and patterns of toothbrushes available to the public. Most of these brushes, according to the buyer, were recommended by dentists. There are long head, short head, soft badger, all grades of hardness of natural bristle and similarly with plastic fibres. Some brushes seem to be quite inappropriate for tooth cleaning, others would appear to be not only ineffective but harmful. How does it happen that all these have claims to dentists' recommendation?

The reasons for the great toothbrush mix-up are many, but have never been adequately discussed in professional circles.

1. Toothbrush design and construction has changed over the years, but, in spite of this, many dentists have remained 'faithful' to their original concepts.

2. Our attitude to 'cleaning' has changed. We consider attention to plaque and gingivae more important than removal of food debris, and enamel polishing or 'whitening'.

The Nylon Bristle Fallacy

Many dentists still believe and staunchly defend their long-held view that *nylon bristle* is harmful and that the use of natural bristle is essential. At the present time this concept is erroneous and is a relic of a genuinely held concern about the quality of nylon a quarter of a century ago. (*Fig.* 19.)

If we observe the brushing methods of a large number of people a surprising number of important facts come to light.
1. Most people wet the brush under a running cold tap before loading with dentifrice.
2. Brushing goes on until the toothpaste has formed so much foam in the mouth that it then becomes necessary to spit and rinse.

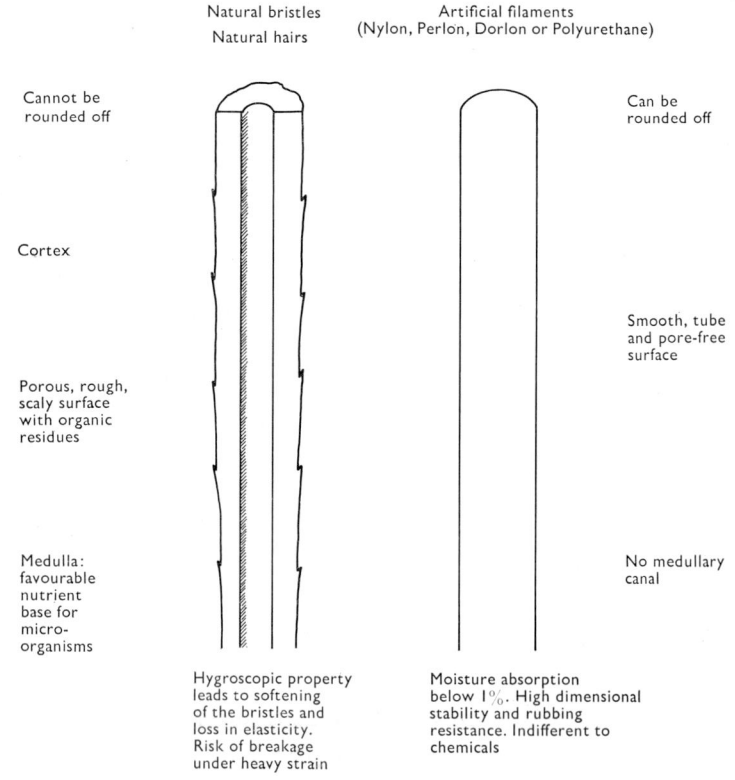

	Natural bristles Natural hairs	Artificial filaments (Nylon, Perlon, Dorlon or Polyurethane)	
Cannot be rounded off			Can be rounded off
Cortex			
			Smooth, tube and pore-free surface
Porous, rough, scaly surface with organic residues			
Medulla: favourable nutrient base for micro-organisms			No medullary canal
	Hygroscopic property leads to softening of the bristles and loss in elasticity. Risk of breakage under heavy strain	Moisture absorption below 1%. High dimensional stability and rubbing resistance. Indifferent to chemicals	

Fig. 19. Comparison between natural and artificial toothbrush filaments. (From Riethe, 1974.)

At this point, however, at which little has been achieved in brushing around all the teeth, most brushers do not continue brushing after this initial rinsing of the mouth. Few ever reload the brush and start again. However, a high percentage constantly wetted the brush at short intervals during brushing. The effect of the initial and/or continuous brush wetting action is to make natural bristles soft and soggy. For this reason the majority of toothbrushes sold in this country were of the 'hard' or 'extra hard' type. But during the days before nylon, the extra hard brush became, after its soaking, something like a soft or soft medium.

When nylon bristled brushes were developed initially, the manufacturers, of course, followed the same hardness formula as was apparently desired by the mass of the population. But man-made fibre was much less moisture absorbent and therefore when wetted as usual by the brusher it did *not* soften but remained hard, or extra hard. The gingivae (and even enamel) were often damaged and at that time nylon bristles acquired a disrepute. Of course, this should have been referred only to the hardness of the brush.

Eventually multitufted plastic filaments, which did not require softening, were introduced and are superior to natural bristle for the following reasons:

1. Plastic bristles can be quality and size controlled to very fine limits. We can make what we want to precise measurements.
2. Plastic bristles are potentially cleaner than natural bristles as they do not absorb fluids and organisms as readily.
3. Natural bristles take longer to dry than the plastic. Thus, if a dry brush is required a twice-daily brusher needs at least two brushes.

In view of the foregoing it is interesting to note that there are strongly supported campaigns in Germany and France to forbid the manufacture and sale of 'natural' bristle toothbrushes.

The Fallacy of the Soft Badger Brush

This was (and still is, surprisingly) recommended by dentists to patients who complained that 'brushing makes my gums bleed'. The badger brush is recommended to 'prevent further traumatizing of the gingivae'. The gingivae rarely bleed with the badger brush because its so gentle action achieves nothing at all. This actually fits in well with the brushing philosophy of most of the population (until now) who brush as a built-in reflex—part of one's cleanliness habits. No account is taken of whether anything is achieved in the way of plaque control: the aim is to do their 'daily duty' and to feel the 'fresh peppermint taste'.

If the patient's gums bleed when brushing, then one should find out why. If the reason is gingivitis associated with plaque (as it usually is) then careful training in brushing is necessary with the appropriate brush ('medium' could be used—*see later*) and the patient told to brush in spite of the bleeding. This will get better if particular attention is paid to brushing these inflamed areas.

The Fallacy of the Round-ended Filaments

Many toothbrush manufacturers (and also dentist researchers) show enlarged photographs of plastic bristles accompanied by a frightening story of how the simply cut bristles have roughened ends which will damage the teeth and gums, whereas the recommended rounding off of the ends is safer and healthier. (Sometimes this is called 'rondating', a term used by one manufacturer.)

If the dentist considers this to be of significance he should specify rounded end bristle brushes. It would, however, be of great interest if he could substantiate this belief by demonstrating actual damage caused by non-rounding off. The truth is that all non-rounded bristles become smoothed very quickly in use. This is similar to the use of a new comb, the teeth of which often feel very rough and scratchy on the scalp on first use, but subsequently are quite smooth (and the scalp is probably more sensitive than the gingiva).

The Choice of Toothbrush

Desirable qualities:
1. Man made (controllable) filaments—generally 0·008–0·011in.
2. Therefore medium or medium soft.
3. Short head (about 1 in)—straight handled—about 6 in total length.
4. Straight trim.
5. Multitufted.
6. But all the above qualities are relatively insignificant in relation to the essential quality—to be able to remove plaque from the teeth.

The type found to be most satisfactory is a multitufted plastic filament brush. Here many fine filaments are packed closely in each tuft and the latter are placed close together so that good coverage of the tooth surface and embrasures is afforded.

British Standard (1979) BS 5757

Adult	Youth	Child
Extra soft (1)	Extra soft (1)	Extra soft (1)
Soft (2)	Soft (2)	Soft (2)
Medium (3)	Medium (3)	Medium (3)
Hard (4)	—	—
Examples:		Examples:
Sensodyne Gentle (1)		Wisdom 'Mouthmaster' Junior (1)
Wisdom 'Mouthmaster' (2)		Gibbs Junior (2)
Boots Oral Hygiene (3)		Wisdom Junior (3)
'Smokers' (4)		

The current British Standard (1979) BS 5757 classifies brushes, according to their length and width, into brushes suitable for adult, youth or child. There is no hard bristle brush approved for youth or child.

This new standard has initiated a number of changes in the texture or hardness of toothbrushes which were hitherto assessed as soft or soft/medium. Some confusion as to the choice exists at present because of the uncertainty between the use given by different manufacturers to the terms soft or medium. However, the effect of the new standard seems to be that the too fine filament diameters (0·007 in, etc.) criticized in the previous edition of this book have now been changed to thicker and more acceptable filament diameters around 0·01 in.

For the generally taught 'roll' brushing technique the medium seems to be satisfactory and acceptable to the patient. For vibratory brushing techniques (such as is recommended in the Bass method), the softer brush is more satisfactory. As the tufts are meant to vibrate in the gingival crevice the dentist may feel that smooth ends are essential. In fact most of the larger manufacturers round off the ends anyway. The hitherto frequently recommended very soft brushes had filament diameters of 0·007 in or less. There was some difficulty in encouraging general and continual use of these because patients did not like the 'too soft' feel of these brushes. As mentioned above this has now been changed with the introduction of the new standard. Patients will, however, continue uncomplainingly with brushes where the filaments are slightly firmer. It would seem to be a waste to teach methods which involve the use of brushes we recommend, but which the patients abandon. Brushes such as the Wisdom Mouthmaster would appear to be readily accepted.

Automatic Brushes

Experience of these brushes from the earliest days of their development leads to the conclusion that only continuously powered or rechargeable brushes are really acceptable. Brushes with conventional replaceable batteries suffer from the disadvantage of an immediate lessening of torque from the first day of use.

All the powered brushes which are acceptable in themselves have quite small heads with multitufted filament.

The potential for damage to the tooth substance or gingivae by powered brushes, a point sometimes brought up by dentists, is limited by the fact that no powered brush can exert the same pressure which can be demonstrated by the healthy-limbed manual brusher. The automatic brush would stall before excessive pressure can be exerted. However, in spite of the advertisers' claims, owners of automatic brushes must be carefully taught how to use them effectively. There is no easy way, even with these brushes. The advantage of the powered brush is that it is easier for the less manually dextrous to achieve some sort of result and once reasonable skill is acquired there is a saving in time over manual brushing. The potential disadvantage of these appliances is that the patient can be lulled into believing that all that has to be done is to purchase one of these and everything will be done for him! There would appear to be little difference in effect between automatic brushes which have arc oscillations, reciprocal horizontal movement or a combination of both. Automatic brushes are sold usually with four replaceable brush heads for use by different members of the family. Tests have demonstrated a mixture of saliva and toothpaste on the handles of these brushes and unless strict cleaning and disinfection is carried out each time before use, the sharing of these brushes by different users is not recommended.

It seems that the manufacturer of the most popular automatic toothbrush in the U.K. is likely to withdraw it from the market. In this event it appears that the only alternatively acceptable brush (the Pifco-Broxodent for mains use) will be available. This must be of great concern because the automatic brush is a beneficial aid to many, especially the handicapped. In this respect a mains driven brush could be a problem in areas where convenient electrical outlets may not be available.

Manual v. Automatic Brushing

All patients where possible should be taught initially an effective plaque removal technique with the manual brush. If the patient is manually incapable (or incapacitated) or even too lazy to spend enough time and effort, then an automatic brush may be recommended and demonstrated. Some of those who are able to brush satisfactorily with a manual brush may want to use an automatic. It is just as important in these cases to go over again the patient's technique with the new brush.

TOOTHBRUSHING METHODS

Although it would be a desirable goal, it is not possible to achieve 100 per cent plaque removal in any but the exceptional patient. We may try very hard to teach various techniques and follow this up with floss instruction and the use of interdental cleaners. Nevertheless, many, if not most, of our patients will fall short of our aims for them. And yet it is important to emphasize here that most of our patients will have a greatly improved gingival condition, some even demonstrating complete resolution of the inflammation. It thus appears obvious that the tissue resistance of most of our patients can cope with a certain amount of residual plaque and this would indicate that the dentist or hygienist should not make a spot judgment on the first visit as to how much training in oral hygiene methods a patient requires. It will be necessary to assess the patient's response over a few visits, and perhaps even after a few months at a recall visit. It will become apparent after a visit or two just how much effort or thoroughness of plaque removal is required from each patient. There are some who will have little gingival inflammation and perhaps no caries, but a notable amount of plaque around the teeth; others will have a minimal amount of adherent micro-organisms and yet may demonstrate acute inflammation. We must therefore modify our approach to each patient depending on the reaction observed.

It must be stressed to the teacher of oral hygiene that terms such as 'correct (or incorrect) brushing' should not be used. There is no right or wrong way to brush the teeth. The result is more important than the method. Therefore, if a patient declares that he can remove plaque and debris using a method of his own, and can show that this method is effective, we would be wrong to insist that he cleans his teeth *our* way. We are therefore concerned with *effective* brushing. Patients often say, 'But my teeth can't be dirty, I brush 20 times a day'. The reply to this remark is, 'It's like having 20 tickets to a lottery. They are all wasted except the one that wins.'

A purely mechanical demonstration of toothbrushing is doomed to failure with most patients. It is necessary to explain to the patient just why he or she is being asked to carry out procedures which are sometimes quite difficult and also time-consuming. The explanation should not just be a general one, but should relate to the patient's problem and be an actual part of the presentation.

Motivation
The nature of plaque and its adhesion to the tooth is carefully explained. The role played in caries and periodontal disease is outlined. At this stage the patient, without having had any toothbrush demonstration, should have been motivated.

Education
The fact that there is not one single 'right' way to brush is emphasized. The right way is any one of a number of different methods which will suit the particular patient.

At this stage the teeth are painted with a disclosing solution and the plaque adhering to the teeth is pointed out to the patient. This indicates the areas which have been missed during home brushing up to now. The plaque is gently scraped off a tooth with the side of a probe to demonstrate how easy it is to remove mechanically.

A suitable brush is selected for the patient and he is told that this is his brush which will be sealed up and kept for training at every visit. Therefore, it is advisable to purchase brushes which are supplied in containers which can be reclosed. (Such a brush, for example, is Oral B 40, or Wisdom Mouthmaster.)

Demonstration

The patient is asked to bring the brush which has up to the present been used at home, but not to buy a new one. It is examined for suitability and the patient is then asked to demonstrate completely how the usual brushing is carried out. It should be explained that as complete a brushing as usual is desired. It is of help to set a stop watch at the start. After observing the patient's routine the time to completion is announced (this is usually of the order of 20–30 seconds, although the brusher often insists that he has taken 2 minutes!).

Errors in brushing, areas omitted, lack of organized method are pointed out. An almost constant error is that patients wet the toothbrush before starting. They should be told that this is an incorrect thing to do, and the much worse procedure, the use of hot water, will damage the bristles. Life-size models are used for individual toothbrush demonstration. (Giant size models are not advised unless demonstrating to a large class.)

Each quadrant is divided into three areas, posterior, middle and anterior, and for brushing purposes these are further subdivided into buccal/labial side and lingual or palatal side (*Fig.* 20). The patient is recommended to brush each of these six areas with 8 strokes of the brush—thus making a total of 48 strokes for each quadrant or approximately 200 strokes for a complete mouth. It has been found that, as noted above, the patient has little concept of time taken for brushing but can readily count 200 strokes. Furthermore, the strokes relate to specific areas of the mouth while, even if say a timer is provided (e.g. egg timer), there is no guarantee that the patient will brush any more methodically.

There are many brushing methods. The dentist or hygienist should not overcomplicate by using too many different techniques, but should be able to demonstrate at least two methods (*Figs.* 21, 22).

The 'Roll' Technique

Effective toothbrushing techniques are not easily acquired by the average patient. Therefore exotic and overcomplicated manoeuvres should be avoided. Perhaps most widely taught (routinely) is the 'roll' method although this still offers difficulties to those who lack manual dexterity, patience, or who have limited wrist movement. The brush is placed on the first of our twelve designated sectors of the

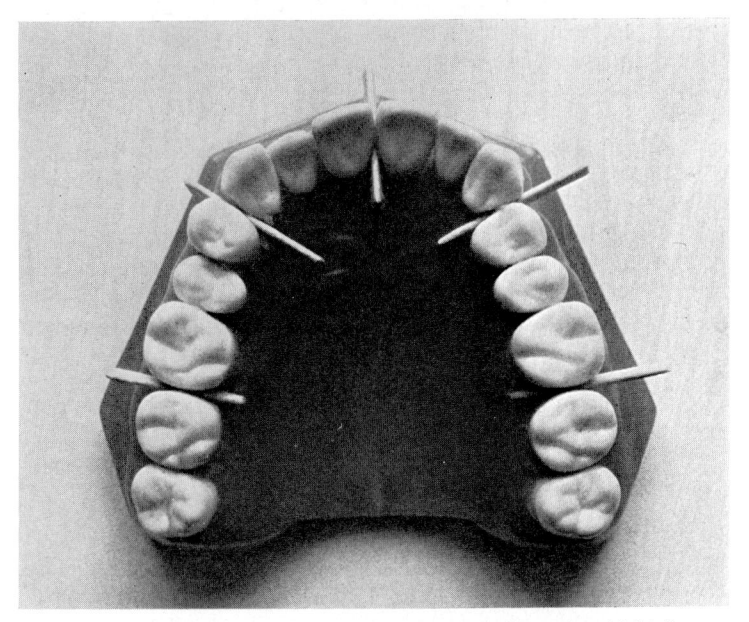

Fig. 20. Division of jaw into 12 brushing areas (lingual and labial). Each area is brushed completely before going on to the next.

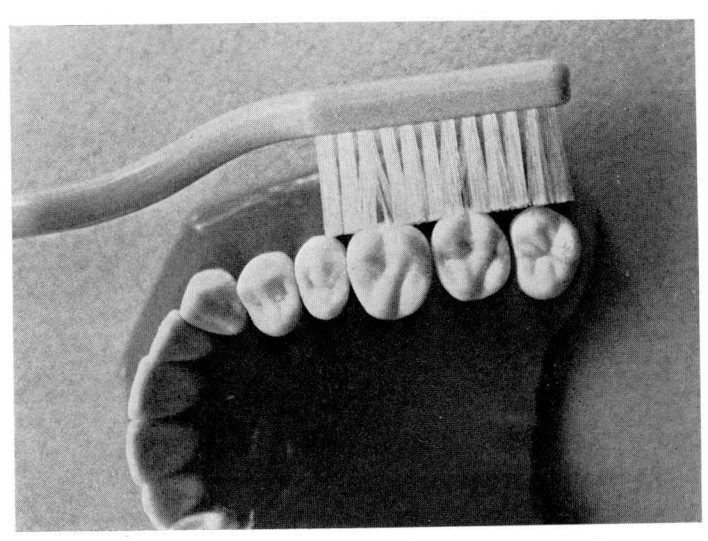

Fig. 21. This placement is incorrect. Here the tips of the bristles press against the teeth but cannot adapt to the shape of the teeth and therefore do not enter the embrasures. It matters not whether the patient brushes up and down or across with this placement. There would be the same lack of effect and potential for damage.

jaw with the bristles on the alveolar mucosa pointing away from the occlusal surface. The side of the bristles press against the attached gingiva and sulcus area. The bristles are then rolled across the gingiva toward the occlusal keeping the sides of the bristles pressed firmly against the tissues (they should appear to blanch) and with many of the bristles sweeping through the embrasures. This stroke is repeated eight times in each region. Assuming that the buccal area was brushed, this is followed by the lingual and repeated around the whole arch. The occlusal surfaces are then brushed with a to-and-fro action. The emphasis in all the brushing is that the brush should be used as a broom to sweep, not as a scrubbing brush to scour. The

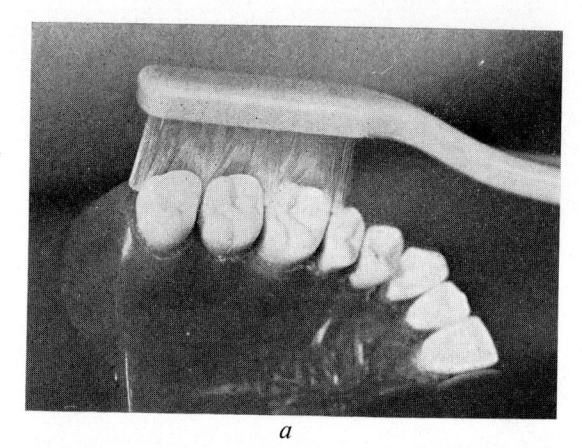

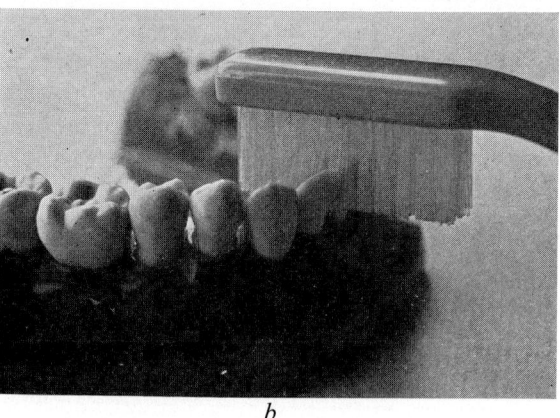

Fig. 22. *a*, Correct placement of brush to adapt to shape of teeth and gingivae. *b*, The lower lingual region is often difficult to brush effectively. The 'split bristles' method shown here is useful —the patient may bite down on the back of brush.

brush is often held vertically for the lingual surfaces of the upper and lower incisor teeth.

The Bass Technique

This is one of the techniques which has become more popular and is dependent on the use of fine plastic multitufted brushes. The brush is applied in the same section by section pattern as previously but with the bristle direction at an angle of 45° to the long axis of the teeth and pointing toward the gingival sulcus. The bristles in fact are made to enter the sulcus and the brush rotated firmly in a small circle without moving the bristle ends from the crevice. In this way the gingival areas of the tooth and the 'pockets' are cleaned. The action is repeated in adjacent areas following the previously described pattern. Some dentists advocate a to-and-fro motion of the bristles in the sulcus area instead of the circular motion. There would appear to be little to choose between the two actions. The lingual areas of the anterior teeth are brushed using the same action but holding the brush head vertically.

The Charters Technique

This is nowadays not used so often as the Bass method and consists of a substantially similar action except that the brush is placed with the bristles pointing occlusally at an angle of 45°, i.e. there is no action of bristle in the gingival sulcus but the vibrating motion concentrates on cleaning the proximal embrasures.

These various methods should not be taught to the patients indiscriminately but the patient's ability to achieve successful plaque removal with the simplest methods should first be evaluated and here differences in tooth alignment, arch form and size, inclination and manual ability may bring about modification in teaching methods. This emphasises the need for personal 'one-to-one' training and the disadvantages of group 'teach-ins'.

Assessment

After each demonstration the patient is asked to brush his own teeth similarly, and the dentist or hygienist may help by placing the patient's brush in the correct position and helping to guide the wrist or hand action. Following this disclosing agents are used and the amount of residual plaque is demonstrated.

A similar procedure is adopted on the following visit approximately one week later, with the disclosed plaque indicating areas which have been overlooked.

Further training is given and it is common for sufficient ability and control to take three to four visits to achieve.

Dentifrices

Although the removal of debris and plaque from the tooth surfaces and gingivae is almost entirely a mechanical one, the importance of a good dentifrice should not be minimized. A report (Consumers' Association, 1974) on dentifrices by an independent non-dental organization was widely publicized as proclaiming that toothpastes were unnecessary as it was 'the brush that did the cleaning'. The readers were also advised to buy the cheapest toothpaste they could get (preferably fluoride containing) and the bargain offers of the local supermarket were recommended.

As dentists and professional advisers we should be more responsible. Our patients expect a little more advice than 'use the one which has the taste that you prefer' or 'use the cheapest you can get'. However, the most recent report from the same organization (Consumer's Association, 1980) in an excellent article 'Caring for the Teeth', gives useful lists of brushes, toothpastes and other aids to oral hygiene.

While we need not necessarily choose one particular brand to recommend to our patients, it is sensible to name two or three which we believe to be safe and useful, and which are believed to have a constantly maintained formulation. One of the dangers of recommending 'supermarket toothpastes' is that they may be 'own brand' products made by unknown manufacturers and sometimes sold on a temporary basis while they are profitable or popular. Without the name of a reputable manufacturer, whose existence depends on maintaining a hard-won and expensively earned public acceptance, the product can be dropped or its formula changed to a more profitable one. As most 'ethical' dentifrice manufacturers now have a medical product licence, it might be that one should confine recommendation of a toothpaste to one which has such a licence.

The dentifrices which are usually worth recommending purely from a therapeutic standpoint are those which contain fluoride compounds, and have been developed and marketed after careful research and testing.

Special Purpose Dentifrices

Some patients who have sensitive cervical areas on their teeth may benefit from the use of desensitising pastes such as Sensodyne or Emoform (Thermodent). Although many patients state that they have been advised to use these pastes to treat gingivitis or periodontitis, there is no justification for such a recommendation. The only possible value for such dentifrices is in the symptomatic treatment of sensitivity of dentine—not gingivae. Before treating painful areas in this manner a thorough investigation into more definitive causes should be carried out.

When these pastes are used, the patient should be instructed to brush with a small amount on a toothbrush—as they would with a 'normal paste' and then to follow up with a little of the paste rubbed with a finger into the sensitive areas.

OTHER CLEANSING DEVICES

Dental Floss

Dental floss may be either waxed or unwaxed. A double width floss, Dentotape is probably easiest for patients to handle. There is at present a vogue for unwaxed floss because it is said that in use

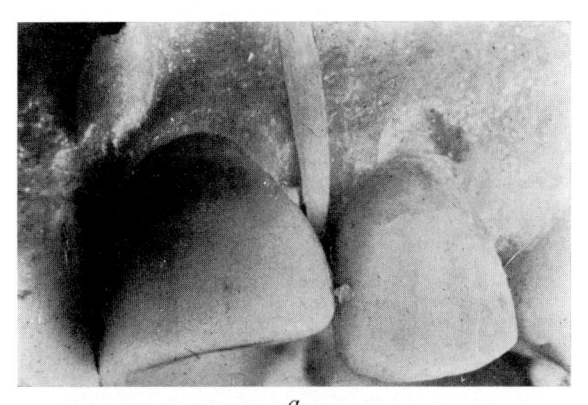

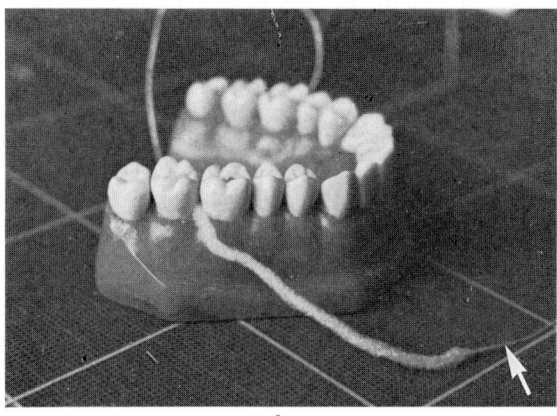

Fig. 23. *a*, Dentotape—the flat wide floss is particularly safe on the gingiva. *b*, Superfloss. The stiffer thin portion (arrowed) is useful for passing under contact points or fixed bridges. The thicker portion is then an excellent plaque remover. The disadvantage of Superfloss is that it comes in separate pieces requiring bulky packaging.

PREVENTIVE DENTISTRY

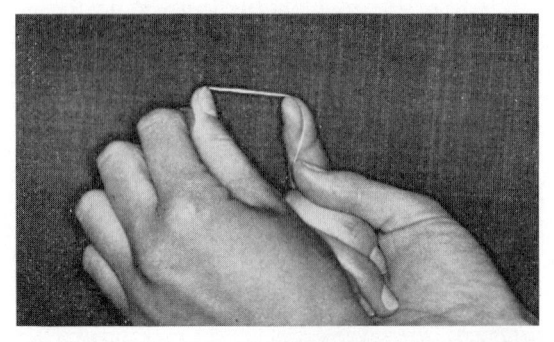

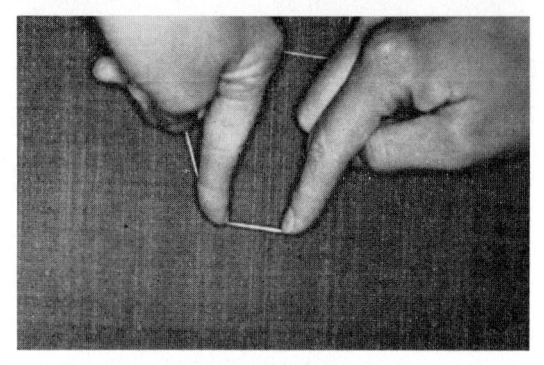

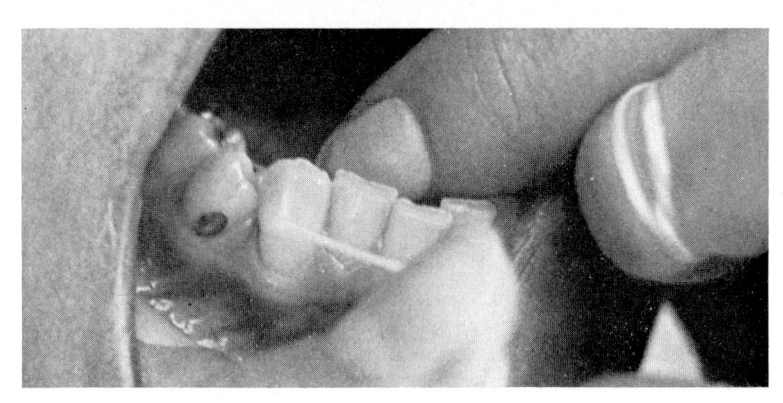

Fig. 24. Using floss: *a*, Holding a loop in position for the upper teeth of left side. *b*, Finger position of loop for lower teeth. *c*, The floss is wrapped around the tooth.

strands open and trap plaque and debris, and hence clean the interdental spaces better. The waxed floss has been used for generations with satisfactory results but in general few patients persevere with the use of either type. Whereas the average patient accepts the use of a toothbrush as part of the daily routine, flossing is not so naturally accepted and considerable difficulty is experienced in handling it. Even if the technique is apparently mastered, enquiry subsequently among our patients has revealed that too many give up after all too short a period.

Technique of Flossing

Careful demonstration is always necessary. Written instructions are useful only after there has been practical training and practice in handling. It has been found easier to cut off a six inch length of floss and tie the ends together to form a loop. This is then held as in *Fig. 24a* between left thumb and right index finger in order to clean the upper left quadrant. The fingers are reversed for the right quadrant. The loop is held as in *Fig. 24b* for the lower teeth. The floss is held taut between the fingers and is gently worked from the occlusal through the contact point down to the gingival crevice where if possible it is slid along the tooth surface just under the crevice and the two hands are brought as near together as possible, thus wrapping the floss around half the circumference of the tooth. In this position the floss is gently drawn occlusally while being kept firmly against the tooth surface. The action is repeated and then the surface of the neighbouring tooth across the embrasure is similarly treated. The patient is instructed to clean all the proximal surfaces changing grip as indicated. Where it is not possible to introduce the floss through a contact point (e.g. soldered contacts of bridge pontics or splints) the material is passed under the contact using a floss threader (Nupons, Zon, etc).

The patients usually have even more difficulty handling unwaxed floss and it is very doubtful whether any supposed advantage will outweigh the difficulties encountered, or will bring measurable benefits except to the floss salesmen. Hill, Levi and Glickman (1973) demonstrated that there were no significant differences in reduction of interdental plaque and interdental gingival inflammation produced by toothbrushing, and toothbrushing followed by the use of floss, either waxed or unwaxed. There are many flossing devices on the market but none is recommended because they are no easier to handle then the floss itself (*see* Chapter 5).

Wood Sticks (Fig. 25)

Many patients will fairly readily take to the use of wood sticks

PREVENTIVE DENTISTRY

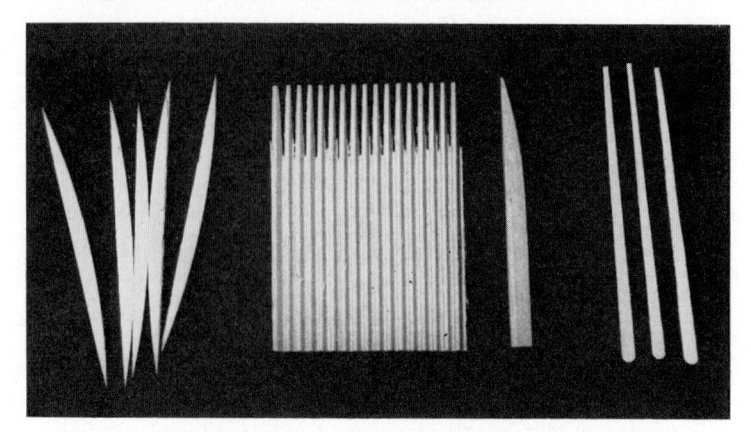

Fig. 25. Different makes of wood sticks. The firmest are the Portia (toothpicks) on the extreme right. For this reason they surprisingly need fairly wide embrasures between the teeth, because they do not compress. Probably the most acceptable sticks today are the Sanodents (double ended), shown at left.

(Sanodents, etc. *see* Appendix 1). These, together with other interdental cleaners of measurable dimensions, should be recommended only where there is sufficient interdental space not filled by gingival tissue. Care is necessary in teaching the use of wood sticks. They should not be used as toothpicks, which is what the patients will tend to do but the stick should be inserted into the embrasure, pointed end first, with the stick at an angle of 45° to the long axis of the tooth, and the sharp edge of the stick away from the gingiva. The stick is rubbed about 12 times in each space with the tip pointing coronally. A methodical approach should be emphasized, that is, the patient should start from a fixed point in the mouth and work round the mouth back to the same point. In fact there should be some order about using the sticks so that no space is missed out. There may be some difficulty in reaching spaces in the posterior part of the mouth, and other devices or techniques may have to be employed. The Portia type of wood sticks (in fact the original idea of toothpicks) are quite inexpensive and may be sufficient for some patients but because they are made of hard wood and do not compress in use, surprisingly they require a little more space than the more compressible Stimudents type of stick.

Interdental Brushes (*Figs.* 26, 27)

The Halex Interspace brush, or the Wisdom Spacemaster (*see Fig.* 26) have the advantage that they will reach the posterior areas easily and patients do not often have difficulty in their use. They have the added advantage of being reasonably inexpensive. It is also possible to clean the embrasures from both lingual and labial aspects of the jaws, other small brushes may be disposable and attached to metal handles by a screw ring (Perio-aid, Perio-pak). They are usually expensive—the bottle-washing type of brush does however remove plaque from the posterior teeth very easily; and a similar brush which can be employed, is the small type of brush which is marketed for cleaning the blades of electric shavers. All are used by entering the embrasures at the same angle as recommended with the wood sticks.

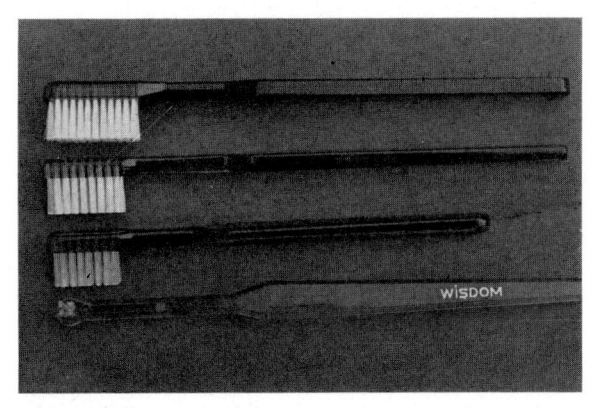

Fig. 26. A modern series of brushes produced in three sizes: fourth row, adult; third row; adult; junior. All in soft/medium nylon with straight trim.

Gauze Strips (*Fig.* 28)

If the spaces between the teeth are wide, the proximal surfaces of the teeth may be cleaned by half inch gauze strips (ribbon gauze would be ideal).

Polishing Cloths

Polishing cloths may be used (thin towelling cut to the shape of the fingers, and sometimes sewn to an average shape by dental staff in possible unoccupied moments) to polish the surfaces of all teeth before brushing. However, this would seem to be a further complication for the already burdened patient but may be reserved as a special armamentarium for the difficult case, e.g. the handicapped child, and here it may be much easier for the mother or other attendant to use a cloth than a brush.

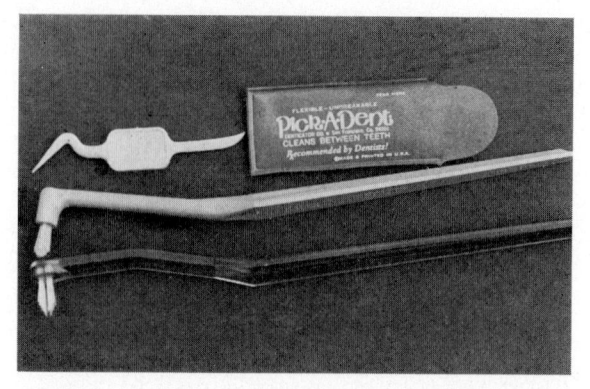

PREVENTIVE DENTISTRY

a

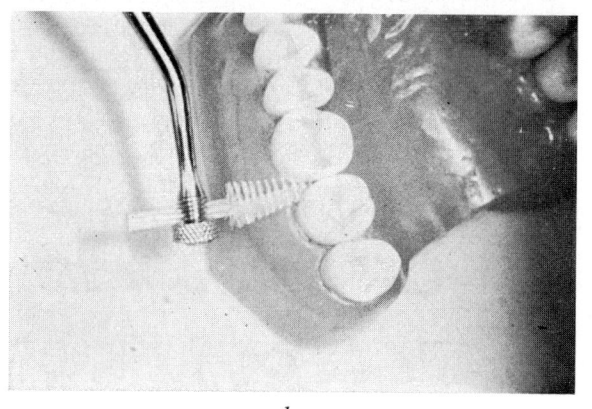

b

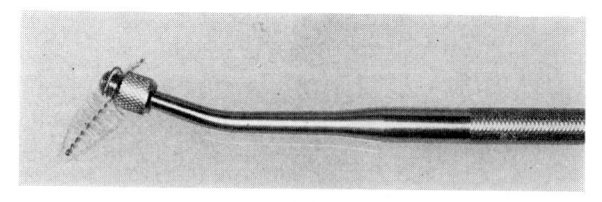

c

Fig. 27. *a*, Some of the current interdental cleaners. From the top: plastic Pick-a-Dent (J. & S. Davis); Interspace (Halex); Spacemaster (Wisdom). *b*, Crescent Perio-pak interdental brush. Note that the free end of the brush is covered with a plastic guard, whereas the Butler type (*c*) has a dangerous wire protrusion which is difficult to avoid.

DENTAL PLAQUE AND ITS CONTROL

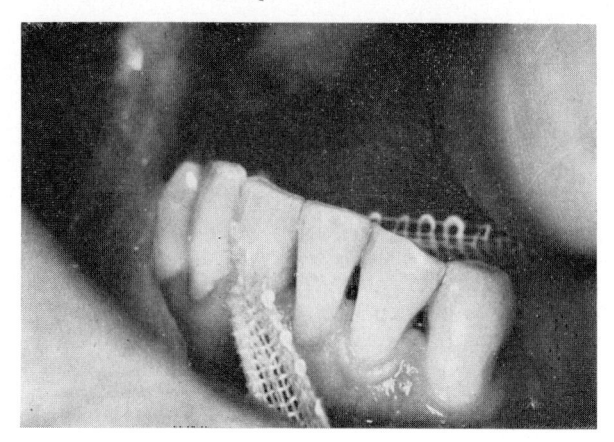

Fig. 28. Gauze strips may be very satisfactory if the spaces are wide enough.

Tongue Cleaning

In some mouths the tongue may play a part in the maintenance of oral infection and this may be noticeable in cases of halitosis. This may be associated with stagnation around the teeth and tongue inactivity may be one factor in both accumulations. We have noticed that many heavy smokers, especially of pipes, have diminished tongue activity perhaps because of initial burning of the tip and then later of lessening tip sensitivity. Tongue activity returns to normal about three months after cessation of smoking. Tongue deposits may be removed by the use of a toothbrush or perhaps with a lesser tendency to cause retching by the use of a tongue scraper. (*Fig.* 29.)

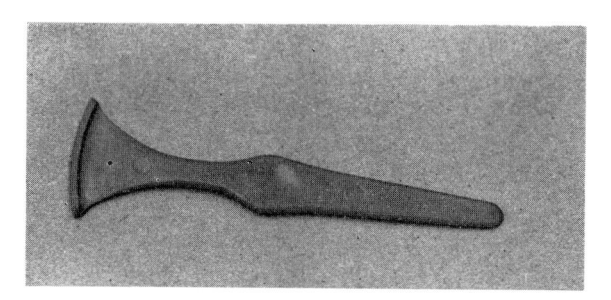

Fig. 29. Tongue scraper specially made for the purpose. However a toothbrush will usually be adequate.

REFERENCES

American Dental Association Council on Dental Materials and Devices (1974). Withdrawal of acceptance of Water Pik oral irrigation device. *J. Am. Dent. Assoc.* **89,** 1178.
Arnim S. S. (1963) The use of disclosing agents for measuring tooth cleanliness. *J. Periodontol.* **34,** 227.
Axelsson P. and Lindhe J. (1974) The effect of a prevention programme on dental plaque, gingivitis and caries in schoolchildren. Results after one and two years. *J. Clin. Periodont.* **1,** 126.
Axelsson P. and Lindhe J. (1978) The effect of controlled oral hygiene procedures on caries and periodontal disease in adults. *J. Clin. Periodont.* **5,** 133–151.
Brasch S. V., Lazarou J., Van Abbe and Forrest J. O. (1969) The assessment of dentifrice abrasivity in vivo. *Br. Dent. J.* **127,** 119.
Consumers' Association (1974) Report on Dentifrices. *Which?* February, p. 36.
Consumers' Association (1980) Caring for Teeth. *Which?* April, pp. 249–254.
Hill H. C., Levi P. A. and Glickman I. (1973) The effects of waxed and unwaxed dental floss on the interdental plaque accumulation and interdental health. *J. Periodontol.* **44,** 411–413.
Horowitz H. S. and Lucye H. S. (1966) A clinical study of stannous fluoride in a prophylaxis base and as a solution. *J. Oral Ther.* **3,** 17.
Kanai S. (1966) The effect of burnishing on the margins of occlusal amalgam fillings. *Acta Odontol. Scand.* **24,** 47, 53.
Kieser J. B. and Wade A. B. (1976) The use of food colourants as plaque disclosing agents. *J. Clin. Periodont.* **3,** 200–207.
Löe H. and Schiott C. R. (1970) The effect of mouthrinses and topical application of chlorhexidine on the development of dental plaque and gingivitis in man. *J. Periodont. Res.* **5,** 79.
Löe H. and Silness J. (1963) Periodontal disease in pregnancy I. *Acta Odontol. Scand.* **21,** 533.
Massler M. (1969) Teenage cariology. *Dent. Clin. North Am.* **13,** 412.
Messing J. J. and Ray G. R. (1972) *Operative Dental Surgery.* London, Kimpton.
Riethe P. (1974) The quintessence of mouth hygiene. Berlin, Quintessence.
Schmid M. O. (1980) The maintenance phase of dental therapy. *Dent. Clin. North Am.* **24,** 389.
Silness J. and Löe H. (1964) Periodontal disease in pregnancy II. Correlation between oral hygiene and periodontal condition. *Acta Odontol. Scand.* **22,** 121.

CHAPTER 4

CONTROL OF THE COMMON DENTAL DISEASES

PART 1: PREVENTION OF CARIES

FLUORIDES IN THE PREVENTION OF DENTAL CARIES

IT has been stated earlier that primary prevention, i.e. protecting against the onset of disease, is far superior to the hitherto practised treatment of incipient disease by drilling and filling. The smallness of a filling gives one no assurance that the margins will not undergo microleakage, whatever the material. Someone once described all filling margins as coming within a classification of: (*a*) Poor, (*b*) Poorer, (*c*) Poorest!

There are basically four factors involved in the initiation of dental caries:

1. The susceptibility of the tooth surface to acid attack.
2. Plaque attached to the tooth surface.
3. The bacterial activity in the plaque.
4. Carbohydrate ingested into the plaque.

The interaction of these factors is illustrated by the simplified equation:

$$\text{Bacteria} + \text{Sucrose} \overset{\text{Plaque}}{=} \text{Acid} + \text{Susceptible tooth surface} = \text{Caries}$$

It would appear that elimination of any one of these would diminish or prevent onset of caries. The prevention of plaque formation on the tooth surface would give a considerable measure of control of bacterial population and would also decrease the ability of the sucrose to be maintained in tooth contact. The control of plaque is discussed elsewhere, but it always creates the dilemma that the patient's maximum co-operation is involved, just as it is if carbohydrate limitation is attempted. Increasing the resistance of the tooth surface enamel against acid products remains the most important means at present which can control dental caries without placing too great a demand on the patient. Heifetz and Suomi (1973) state that many of the measures now advocated for the control of dental disease may be suitable for highly motivated patients but they question whether they are applicable to a wide-scale public health programme. They say that merely possessing a correct attitude is not the same as taking the necessary action. The capability to induce mass behaviour change through public health programmes is still not available. When asked how successful we have been in changing the habits of the population in regard to sweets and in-between snacks, we are bound to answer, 'Not at all'. They go on to say that the greatest 'pay-off' in terms of wide-scale control of oral disease exists in capitalizing as heavily as possible on preventive measures which by-pass individual co-operation or keep it at best to a minimum.

CARIES SUSCEPTIBILITY TESTS

The dentist or his staff may use tests such as the Snyder test to illustrate the existing condition of caries susceptibility in the mouth. The test (and there are many modifications of it) uses a colour indicator to show the amount of acid formed by micro-organisms in a carbohydrate medium and thus measures the quantity of micro-organisms which are capable of acting on carbohydrates to convert them to acids. It is doubtful whether the claimed degree of relationship between actual caries activity and the test results can be relied upon, but it has been suggested that anyway the tests may be used as a patient education aid in motivation for sucrose reduction. This writer, however, has some reservations regarding the ethics of using such tests (which may be costly in materials and time) which have a doubtful diagnostic value but are substitute teaching aids. However, those who may be interested may purchase test kits and instructions from some dental supply houses.

Another factor to be noted is host resistance to the carious process. Much work is being carried out on caries immunization. Animal experiments have shown much promise. The translation of such results to humans may be a problem of acceptability by the public may be an even greater problem. However, the results of such research must be of enormous benefit in increasing our knowledge of the mechanisms of their defence against caries. It may be that subjects with natural immunity have a higher concentration of secretory immunoglobulin (IgA) in the saliva. This appears to alter (probably by 'coating') the cariogenic bacteria so that they cannot produce harmful acids.

Protective factors may occur in the teeth themselves but this is much more difficult to investigate.

To summarize, the dentist's or hygienist's attitude to the possibility of changing any patient's diet should not be too optimistic. If it were universally and immediately possible the problem of dental disease would be solved overnight. However, the dental team should not under-estimate what can be achieved by enthusiasm, constant repetition, careful teaching of young patients—the younger the better—and of course parental example.

CONTROL OF THE COMMON DENTAL DISEASES—PART 1
FLUORIDATION OF WATER SUPPLIES

The resistance of the enamel surface of the tooth to acid attack can be very greatly enhanced by the incorporation of minute amounts of fluoride ion so that the hydroxyapatite crystals become fluoroapatite.

The formation of this solubility resistant form explains the mode of action of fluorides as preventive agents. The fluoride-enriched enamel may be found in the outer layers to the extent of 30–40 μm, with the highest fluoride levels nearest the surface. This would account for the ability of fluorine compounds to act topically, a process of diffusion and exchange taking place at the surface and this is also taking place between the salivary ions and the enamel surface. Thus, there is a two-way passage through the enamel surface 'membrane' but if the fluoride ions are somehow combined with salivary agents to form non-ion soluble compounds or are otherwise lost with similarly lost Ca ions then the resistance of the tooth surface will be decreased. Similarly an increase in salivary F ions from outside sources will tend to increase the flow of ions inwards and hence increase the fluoroapatite content.

In the child, the developing tooth will receive its necessary building materials from the blood plasma and thus the enamel fluorine content will at this point be completely dependent on systemically absorbed fluorine. After tooth eruption maturation of the enamel takes place and there is considerable evidence that a great deal of fluoride uptake is a topical one. Hence it may be assumed that fluoride acts in two complementary ways—by systemic action and by its topical action.

Thus the measure which, in view of the foregoing, brings the greatest benefit in terms of caries control from all aspects is fluoridation of public water supplies, i.e. ensuring an optimum level of 1 ppm of fluoride. An enormous amount of careful research has been carried out for three decades or more on the safety, efficacy and cost of this measure and an overwhelming mass of favourable evidence has been published. Those who may be subjected to anxious questions by members of the public who have been bombarded by objectors are referred to a review published in reply to an attack on fluoridation in a national newspaper (Burt, 1973).

The long-term effects are greatest if the optimum fluoride level in water is available from birth. Children pass to adulthood with an increased number of sound healthy teeth. The total need for restorative dentistry is reduced, and those fillings which are necessary are usually simple.

The dentist in practice may question his connection with fluoridation of water supplies. He must be aware that this measure would make his own work much easier, and combined with his own preventive attitude will bring a new dimension and change to his practice. The dentist and his team should add support to the strenuous efforts being made to introduce the benefits to more and more of the population. The dentist should have access to a large quantity of published material for education of the public and also, if he becomes more involved, for the information of his local authorities.

Regrettably, however, the progress of fluoridation of public water supplies has not been advancing in the past few years owing to strenuous campaigns by limited, but active opponents.

FLUORIDE TABLETS

In the absence of controlled adequate fluoride levels of public water supplies much consideration has been given to the daily supply of fluoride tablets (usually 2·2 mg, giving a fluoride dose of 1 mg daily). Investigations have shown substantial reduction in dental caries with deciduous and permanent dentition when consumption of the tablets has been started early enough. However, it has often been shown that even where tablets are provided without charge there is an eventual 'drop out', with only a small percentage of parents persisting with daily dosage to their children.

In view of the benefits derived from these tablets Davies (1973) strongly recommends that when fluoridation of water is impracticable dentists, doctors and child health clinics should be encouraged to prescribe them. He adds that countries with a national health service should consider including fluoride tablets as a pharmaceutical benefit. An alternative procedure would be to arrange for distribution of the tablets through kindergartens and schools.

When consideration is given to prescribing or distributing tablets it is essential to ascertain the fluoride content of the water supply in the recipient's area of residence. It is not sufficient to base distribution on the known fluoride level of the water in the dentist's area. Dosage should then be adjusted to the known natural fluoride residential level, with of course no tablet prescription when this reaches a level of 1 ppm. The recommended dosage for children under 3 years of age has been reduced as there have been occasional occurrences of (mild) enamel fluorosis. Thus the recommended dose for a child under 2 years of age would be 0·25 mg F which would be ¼ tablet. In view of the difficulty of dividing tablets in this way it is felt that the fluoride paediatric solutions now marketed are more acceptable (*see* Chapter 6).

Mothers should be warned to keep the tablets out of reach of children, to avoid accidental overdosage. For this reason fluoride tablets disguised as sweets are to be deprecated.

TOPICAL FLUORIDES

The dentist newly entering the field of preventive dentistry tends to believe that this part of the text is the real 'meat' of prevention. One hopes that the previous chapters have convinced him that 'putting something on the teeth', whether it be fluorides or fissure sealants, is only a part of the preventive picture. There is abundant literature evaluating the effects of topical fluoride solutions on the teeth. Bernier and Muhler (1966) list 219 references on the effect of various forms of topical fluoride therapy.

The three main fluoride agents are:

1. Sodium fluoride (NaF), usually applied as a 2 per cent solution in distilled water.
2. Stannous fluoride (SnF_2), usually in an 8 or 10 per cent solution.
3. Acidulated phosphate fluoride solution or gel (1·23 per cent fluoride ion).

1. *Sodium Fluoride*

The first report of a clinical study using NaF was made by Bibby in 1944. He used a 0·1 per cent solution and gave three applications which resulted in a caries reduction of 30 per cent after one year. The use of 2 per cent solution was first reported by Knutson and Armstrong in 1943, and since that time there have been many trials with results giving annual caries reductions of up to 69 per cent DMFS (decayed, missing and filled surfaces).

The sodium fluoride is stable but should preferably be kept in a plastic bottle. The 2 per cent solution can be made up conveniently by the local pharmacist and is obviously a readily available and inexpensive product. This is a great advantage.

Technique

In all topical fluoride techniques it is recommended that the teeth be cleaned prior to fluoride application. A harsh abrasive prophylactic paste should be avoided (*see* p. 33) and it is recommended that one of the proprietary fluoride-containing pastes be used or fluoride solution should be added to the paste before use. Dental floss should be passed through the contact points to remove any plaque or debris in the proximal areas.

Following this the teeth are isolated with cotton wool rolls, a quadrant at a time, and a high speed evacuator is placed in position. The cleaned, isolated teeth are dried by further use of the air syringe and the teeth are then constantly wetted with the sodium fluoride for a period of 4 minutes. After each quadrant is completed the patient is allowed to spit and then the other quadrants are completed in turn.

At the termination of the total application the patient is allowed to spit and rinse once only. Average application time is 10 minutes.

The routine use of sodium fluoride 2 per cent would appear to have been largely superseded by the other fluorides but there is no doubt that if no other agent had been introduced we should still be able to obtain very considerable reductions of new caries increments.

There are many conflicting reports showing superiority of one type of fluoride over another, but no consensus of opinion from the various trials can be obtained. The conclusions which can be made are that all the mainly used fluorides do affect considerable reductions in DMFS. The differences between them may be marginal and as each type has its staunch advocates the use of a particular agent is often a matter of individual choice, based on convenience, comparative cost and availability. This will be discussed later.

2. *Stannous Fluoride*

A solution of 10 or 8 per cent in distilled water is applied to the teeth for 2 minutes.

Considerable work was carried out with stannous fluoride by Muhler and his co-workers in Indiana. Their findings suggested a much enhanced effect in caries reduction over sodium fluoride but this has not always been confirmed by other workers. However, the following are some properties of the stannous fluoride solution.

1. It is very active and therefore loses its potency rapidly and must be freshly mixed, therefore, by the dentist or his assistant for each application session.
2. It is claimed that stannous fluoride is more effective in adults than NaF.
3. It seems to have effects even in those areas where there is optimum water fluoridation.
4. It tends to stain incipient carious lesions and there is criticism of the pigmentation produced.
5. There is a metallic taste which some patients find objectionable.
6. Muhler claimed that a single yearly application of 8 per cent stannous fluoride was sufficient to give caries protection.
7. Further studies tend to show that less than the usual 4-minute exposure given with most topical agents will give effective caries reduction. Mercer and Muhler (1964) reported good results with 30-second treatments, while Scola and Ostrom (1968) further reduced the application time to 15 seconds with similar reported success. Shannon (1972) has reported the development of a stable stannous fluoride 0·4 per cent gel (water-free) with glycerin which shows exceptional promise. If this is indeed successful the low stannous fluoride concentration will be much more acceptable from a taste aspect.

Technique for Stannous Fluoride Topical Applications

A stannous fluoride supply can be obtained (in the U.K.) from Oral Hygiene Products (*see* Appendix 1). When this is used in our practice we always make up a 10 per cent solution.

One gram of stannous fluoride crystals is dissolved in 10 ml of distilled water. A 10 ml discarded hypodermic syringe makes a convenient measure for the water which is then added to the crystals which have been poured into a small bottle and the mixture is shaken until there is a clear solution.

The teeth are cleaned and polished as described previously. Cotton rolls are inserted to isolate a quadrant (or sometimes both quadrants on the same side). The solution is applied to the teeth with a cotton tip, keeping the teeth wet continuously for 2 minutes. Dental floss is passed through the contact areas to ensure that they are wetted with the solution. Unwaxed floss is usually recommended but it is doubtful whether this really matters. Each quadrant is similarly treated in sequence.

Time taken on average for complete application is 5 minutes.

Comments

This has been the standard topical fluoride technique of my own practice for the past 20 years, but there is no doubt that the acidulated sodium phosphate solutions or gels are being used currently to a far greater extent.

The quoted disadvantages of the stannous fluoride solutions:

1. The pigmentation of some areas of the teeth.
2. The necessity to mix fresh solutions before treatments.
3. Objections to the taste.

1. Pigmentation (brown or black areas) has never been a cause for anxiety. The staining is associated with incipient areas of caries and indicates arrest of the lesion. It is said to be due to the formation of tin phosphate. Areas which were chalky and soft become brown and *hard*. There is some evidence of remineralization. For the beginner in prevention—who may lack confidence in the ability of topical fluoride solutions to protect the teeth—the evidence of the staining of these incipient lesions demonstrates quite dramatically that a positive effect has occurred. *Intact* enamel does not stain.

2. No difficulty has ever been encountered in preparing fresh stannous fluoride solutions. Very little time is taken with ready to hand materials.

3. The objections to taste vary with different patients. Most children do accept the procedure but some dislike it intensely. However, there is no reason why the stannous fluoride concentration should not be reduced by half or APF gels may be used for those

few who would not tolerate the taste of stannous fluoride. Some advantages of stannous fluoride are the reported high activity of the solution allowing even a 15 or 30 second treatment to be effective. This is important if a child tends to be restless, when a useful application can still be made. Furthermore, because of this it has never been found necessary to use special applicators or trays.

Acidulated Phosphate Fluoride (APF)
Solution or gel

This is usually a commercially available product containing 1·23 per cent fluoride. It is the most widely available topical fluoride agent and it is probably now the most widely used. A 4-minute treatment is advised for each area treated. The gels often have added flavours, e.g. orange, grape, lime.

Technique (*Fig.* 30)

This follows the same pattern as previously described. However, it appears that the 4-minute treatment is rigidly recommended and it

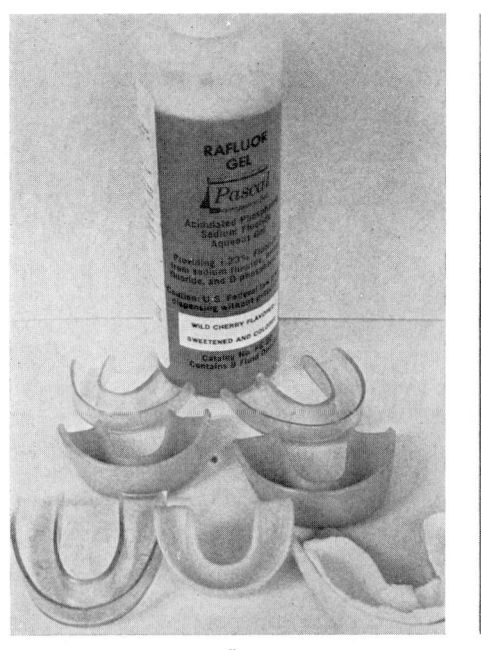

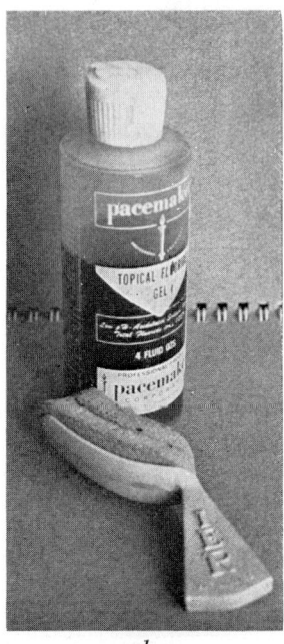

Fig. 30. *a*, Applicators for APF gels or solutions. *b*, Contains a foam material and comes in full or half arch sizes.

is often advised that special applicators be used to hold the gel or solution in place for the required time. In this way either the lower or upper jaw can be completed in one 4-minute period; and with some applicators the whole mouth may be treated at once. *Average application time* 10 *minutes.*

It is difficult to be dogmatic about the superiority of any one of these solutions. The preventive dentist must make his own choice but may well decide for the APF solution or gel mainly because it is readily available from so many dental supply houses and is well advertised. Stannous fluoride is no longer available in the U.K. from the previous suppliers. For a convenient source *see* Appendix 1.

Davies (1973) states that the best results using combination treatment were obtained by using a three point programme: (1) Stannous fluoride prophylaxis paste, followed by (2) Topical application of stannous fluoride, and to advise (3) Home use of a stannous fluoride dentifrice. He estimates that this is probably the most economic community approach (other than water fluoridation).

One's own view is that this is substantially correct and any practice adopting this routine would obtain excellent results in preventing dental caries. In our own practice we have returned to the use of topical stannous fluoride after 2–3 years with APF gels and solutions, although the latter are used for some patients.

Notes for Clinical Practice

1. Topical application of fluoride should be carried out 3 times a year because this is usually made to coincide with school vacations. Parents are taught, 'School holidays means dentist'—this is fundamental to our preventive practice. Thus repeat intervals have a meaning as compared to 6-monthly visits which in the U.K. at least are not related to the school timetable. (To relieve congestion we also relate some visits to 'every half term'.)

2. Topical applications must start with the deciduous teeth and preferably at age $2\frac{1}{2}$–3 years. Again this has been found to be fundamental to preventive practice.

3. Only part of the visit is spent in applying topical agents. A similar amount of time should be spent on instruction or training in dental health care and diet.

There would seem to be some agreement that the effectiveness of topical fluoride treatments is of the order of 30–45 per cent caries reduction.

However, most trials have been necessarily carried out on a limited basis, say over two years, and mostly on children at school, i.e. a captive population. The dentist in practice should be able to improve on the above percentage figures by starting his treatments on the pre-school age children as recommended.

Other Methods of Fluoridation

The practising dentist should be aware of alternative methods for a number of reasons.

1. Patients will question him about them and their efficacy and practicability. He should be able to discuss the pros and cons.
2. It may be that the family live in an isolated area with no possibility of water fluoridation or regular visits to the dentist for preventive attention.
3. Alternative methods may be introduced into the patient's community.

Fluoride Mouth Rinses

There are now many reports of controlled trials which have demonstrated the efficacy of fluoride mouth rinses. Gross and Tinanoff (1977) reported marked reductions of bacteria on enamel with the use of stannous fluoride rinses. Abramson et al. (1978) reported a significant decline in DMF rates in all age groups of children initially age 7, 9, 11 and 13 years using a 0·5 per cent sodium fluoride rinse weekly for 1 minute. An improved oral hygiene state was also noted. Studies have shown that supervised regular rinsing (every week or fortnight) with 0·2 per cent sodium fluoride, stannous fluoride or APF solution will reduce the amount of dental decay.

The principle to be noted here is frequent rinsing with very dilute solutions. This is almost an inverse ratio. Further research continues and a definite method that is generally applicable requires to be formulated. Bearing in mind that mouth rinsing trials may be in progress at some schools the dentists should make enquiries about other sources of fluoride before he himself either provides or prescribes further fluoridation. It is important to monitor the care with which rinsing programmes are supervised. Thus very small children, say under 7, would not be good subjects because of the danger of swallowing much of the solution.

Fluoride in Milk

In view of the slow progress in the implementation of water supply fluoridation there may be some argument in favour of the provision of selective milk fluoridation. Studies have shown some effectiveness but there are a number of counter arguments (such as that the responsibility for protection is thrust back on the parent) and further much more carefully controlled research is required. However, such supply counters one of the arguments of the anti-fluoride lobby, of enforced mass medication.

Fluoride in Pregnancy

Some expectant mothers enquire whether supplements taken before the birth of the child will help in the development of the infant's teeth. There is some conflict as to whether there is any reasonable passage of fluoride ion across the fetal barrier. In the U.S.A. products that claim to prevent decay in babies still unborn are banned as not proved effective. (Also *see* Chapter 6.)

FISSURE SEALANTS

Considerable interest has been aroused by the reported use of sealants in fissures, pits and defects in the enamel surfaces of teeth in order to prevent dental plaque accumulation in these vulnerable areas which could lead to a carious lesion. Although much has now been published about these materials, especially of laboratory trials, the clinical results published have been limited by the short duration of the observations. There is, however, some evidence that *if* the material is correctly applied and *if* it effectively seals the fissures without leakage, then a reduction of fissure caries has been observed over the one or two year periods of the trials.

A great number of dentists who have been involved in prevention, especially on a clinical basis, doubt the true efficacy of, or necessity for, these fissure sealants, and their arguments are based, among others, upon the following reasons:

1. Use of fissure sealants does not eliminate the need for the use of topical fluorides.
2. The fissure sealant, even if effective, protects one surface of the tooth mainly (the occlusal). The other four surfaces at risk (the mesial, distal, buccal and lingual) are dependent on the effect of fluorides and of plaque control by the patient.
3. Many observers experienced in the use of topical fluorides over a number of years, especially with the use of stannous fluoride, do not agree with the advocates of fissure sealants who claim that fluorides are ineffective or of little effect in preventing fissure caries. In this respect Englander (1979) argues that waterborne fluoride does protect occlusal fissures and buccal pits significantly against dental caries, but not to the same extent that it protects proximal and other smooth surfaces. He states that in a recent study of seven cities in five states of the U.S.A. they have found that waterborne fluoride exerted an important anti-caries action on all surfaces recorded. When the mean DMFS scores for 12–15-year-old children in one fluoridated city were compared with those for a similar group in a non-fluoridated city, there was a difference as great as 91 per cent for proximal surfaces and 82 per cent for occlusal sites in favour of the fluoridated city.

It is difficult to find a study in which the effect of fissure sealants has been compared directly to various forms of fluoride application or ingestion in the same group. Therefore, although one accepts the favourable results using sealants as reported by Rock (1974), Horowitz et al. (1974), the review by Boudreau and Jerge (1976) concludes, 'Available evidence demonstrates that sealants are effective in preventing occlusal decay, although studies must be continued for longer periods to provide definite data ... this technique has progressed through various stages of refinement and appears to be *approaching the threshold of acceptability* as a preventive dentistry technique of established value'.

4. Fissure sealants should be applied only to those fissures which are so deep that they are potentially carious but not in fact affected by caries. There is some argument as to whether 'sealing in' caries would be harmful—if the seal were 100 per cent effective this would probably be safe, but in practice one cannot be sure of 100 per cent sealing. The choice of which fissures to seal may involve a considerable exercise of judgement and some forecasting—or even guesswork—at the expense of the patient.

5. Fissure sealants, therefore, must be regarded as applicable where used only for primary caries prevention, whereas topical fluorides, especially of the stannous fluoride type, may be effective in controlling already initiated caries and in the reversal of small lesions.

6. The application of the sealant material is far from simple and the many papers giving examples of loss rates of some sealants exemplify this.

7. One may propose the conflict that could arise with regard to the possibility of this procedure being carried out by other members of the dental team (e.g. dental hygienists). If it is considered acceptable for a first molar to be so treated by acid etch techniques in a possibly difficult situation at the back of the mouth followed by the application of a resin, how can it be considered ethically wrong for the same ancillary worker to do virtually the same procedure on an incisor, say, for an adult and restore a chipped corner or fill an erosion area?

However, the main factor must be that it is costly in time and procedure to use these materials in relation to the benefit obtained, and in the present controversial situation it may not appear justifiable to some to involve patients in the necessarily high fees entailed. There may be commercial pressure to use these materials because they are expensive and therefore more profitable to sell than topical fluorides.

Types of Sealants

At present there are available a number of different commercial sealants. The majority are based on the BIS–GMA resin (which is also the main ingredient of most of the new composite filling materials). There are differences in the way in which the sealants are polymerized or cured (after being placed in position). The material which clinical evidence has to date shown to have better adhesive and sealing qualities is one which does not harden until it is irradiated by high intensity light focused on it from a special lamp. It then polymerizes quickly. The other material hardens by a chemical reaction between the mixed components of the applied paste. There would appear to be some doubt regarding the safety of the unmodified ultraviolet lamp and the use of such lamps unmodified, has been or should have been abandoned.

Adhesion for all these materials is obtained by partly decalcifying the immediately surrounding enamel surface, usually by the use of 50 per cent phosphoric acid or citric acid. The acid etches the surface of the enamel dissolving some of the mineral constituents to a depth of 7–10 μm, and this roughens the surface enabling the fluid sealant to flow into the open pits and on setting there should be a strong bond formed.

If the decision is made to use fissure sealants, the dentist should study very carefully the instructions for use which are issued by the manufacturer of the particular sealant chosen. This advice regarding method of application is likely to be more accurate than any detailed instruction given in this chapter as all the different materials have variations in composition, however slight. The true biologically adhesive glass ionomer cements may be a considerable advance.

SUMMARY
Primary Prevention of Caries

Effective plaque reduction is an important factor in primary caries prevention. The most commonly practised method (see other chapters) and the most generally effective is by the trained use of the toothbrush. Plaque elimination must be a part of prevention in all stages, primary, secondary and tertiary.

It will be difficult to teach the very young child to brush effectively, and before the onset of disease it is beyond the capabilities or desire of the very young child or adolescent to carry out tedious brushing (or flossing) procedures in the expectation of avoiding some disease in the remote future. Thus motivation must be strong and must be combined with the message and training repeated frequently—at all recall visits. However, fluoridation in all its forms is the prime caries preventive agent, taking precedence even over plaque control in the young child.

Secondary Prevention of Caries

With already established caries, whether newly formed and just detectable or gross, perhaps rampant, caries, attention should be paid first of all to the prevention of new cavities forming. The carious tooth should not be finally filled (the cavities can be dressed) until the 'infection' of dental caries is controlled or eliminated. Analogy: it is useless to fill up the holes in the skirting boards without getting rid of the mice. They will just make new holes!

One of the more important aspects of secondary prevention, detecting the early carious lesion, is careful inspection and this often involves the use of X-rays (in the form of bitewings) on a routine basis.

Tooth Defects other than through Caries

Toothbrush abrasion, especially at the vestibular cervical regions of the teeth occurs in connection with overenthusiastic brushing usually with a hard brush. Some abrasive types of toothpastes (or powders) will enhance this effect. Early training in the correct use of the toothbrush will prevent this happening. Once the defects have been incurred there may be sensitivity and this is best treated by a ten-day home rinse programme (2+ minutes per day) with 0·4 per cent stannous fluoride rinse (e.g. Iradicav).

One of the most frequent causes of non-carious tooth tissue loss is through exposure to acids, commonly the intake of acid fruit juices, especially lemons and grapefruit on a regular basis. Patients should be warned of the very considerable enamel dissolution which can occur, and should it not be possible to cease the intake should be instructed in the use of chunky straws or the other methods such as mouth rinsing immediately following intake. (*Fig.* 31.)

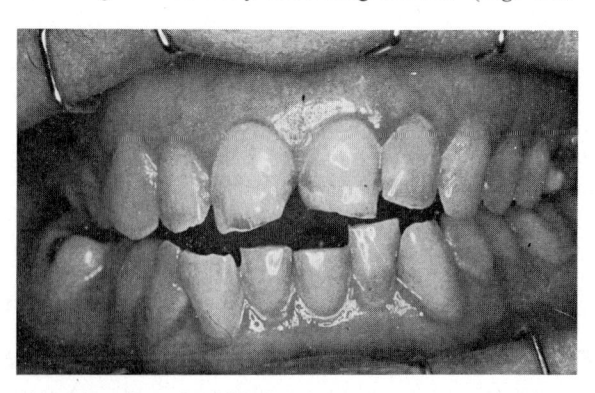

Fig. 31. The effect of acid fruit juices on enamel. Note the highly polished damaged areas after brushing. (By courtesy of Professor A. H. Rowe.)

REFERENCES
Fluorides
Abramson A., Hicks T. W. and Philion J. (1978) Fluoride rinse program. *Can. J. Public Health* **69**, 143–145.
Bernier J. L. and Muhler J. C. (1966) *Improving Dental Practice through Preventive Measures*. St. Louis, Mosby, p. 124.
Bibby, B. G. (1944) Use of fluorine in the prevention of dental caries, II. *J. Am. Dent. Assoc.* **31**, 317.
Burt B. A. (1973) Water fluoridation. *Br. Dent. J.* **135**, 543.
Davies G. N. (1973) Fluoride in the prevention of dental caries—A tentative cost-benefit analysis. *Br. Dent. J.* **135**, 336.
Gross A. and Tinanoff N. (1977) Effect of SnF_2 mouth rinse on initial bacterial colonization of tooth enamel. *J. Dent. Res.* **56**, 1179–1183.
Heifetz S. J. and Suomi J. D. (1973) The control of dental caries and periodontal disease: a fundamental approach. *J. Public Health Dent.* **33**, 2.
Knutson J. W. and Armstrong W. D. (1943) Effect of topically applied sodium fluoride on dental caries experience. *Public Health Rep.* **58**, 1701.
Mercer V. H. and Muhler J. C. (1964) The effect of a 30-second topical stannous fluoride treatment on clinical caries reduction in children. *J. Oral. Ther. Pharm.* **1**, 141.
Murray, J. J. (1976) *Fluorides in Caries Prevention*. Bristol, Wright.
Scola F. P. and Ostrom C. A. (1968) Clinical evaluation of stannous fluoride in naval personnel. *J. Am. Dent. Assoc.* **77**, 594–597.
Shannon I. L. (1972) Dialogue on preventive dentistry. Chicago, March, p. 156.

Fissure Sealants
Boudreau G. E. and Jerge G. R. (1976) The efficacy of sealant treatment in the prevention of pit and fissure dental caries: A review and interpretation of the literature. *J. Am. Dent. Assoc.* **92**, 383–387.
Buonacore M. (1970) Adhesives for pit and fissure caries control. *Dent. Clin. N. Am.* **16**, 693.
Eames W. B. (1972) Pit and fissure sealants. *J. Ga Dent. Assoc.* **46**, 20.
Editorial Comment (1974) *J. Dent.* **2**, 91.
Englander H. R. (1979) Fluoridation protects occlusal areas. *J. Am. Dent. Assoc.* **98**, 11.
Horowitz M. S., Heifetz S. B. and McCune R. J. (1974) Effect of an adhesive sealant in preventing occlusal caries. *J. Dent. Res.* **53** (special issue) 253 abst. 793.
McLean J. W. and Wilson A. D. (1974) Fissure sealing and filling with an adhesive glass ionomer cement. *Br. Dent. J.* **136**, 269.
Parkhouse R. C. and Winter G. B. (1971) The fissure sealant containing methyl and cyanoacrylate as a caries preventive agent. *Br. Dent. J.* **130**, 16.
Rock W. P. (1972) Fissure sealants: results obtained with 2 different sealants after 1 year. *Br. Dent. J.* **133**, 146.
Rock W. P. (1974) Fissure sealants: results of clinical trials. *Br. Dent. J.* **136**, 317.
Williams B., Casson M. H. and Winter G. B. (1974) A clinical study using a new ultra violet light polymerised fissure sealant. *J. Dent.* **2**, 101.

CHAPTER 5

CONTROL OF THE COMMON DENTAL DISEASES

PART 2: PERIODONTAL DISEASE

IF IT were possible to initiate a perfect and rigid individual plaque control then the vast majority of our patients would never have gingivitis or, later, periodontal disease. This is a dream and the discipline involved may be carefully observed by some but becomes too tedious and lacking in urgency for most adolescent patients. There is the eternal problem of giving regular consideration to something that may occur in years ahead. How many people at 18 years of age voluntarily think about saving for a retirement pension maturing at 60?

Very few, if any, patients can ever achieve perfect plaque control. We may demonstrate by cleaning the patient's teeth under the ideal conditions with a good light such as we have in the dentist's office, with brushes, cups, various polishing pastes, strips, tape, etc. Now a disclosing solution is applied. Can we ever swear that there will be no tell-tale red stain somewhere? How can a patient do better under home conditions even if fanatical? Therefore we must accept a varying level of plaque control from each patient.

What level of plaque control is acceptable will depend on our enthusiasm, teaching ability, the patient's skill and interest and the tissue susceptibility. This is the key to the periodontal story.

The prevention of plaque accumulation or its regular removal is, in spite of the foregoing, our best method of avoiding periodontal disease, and therefore the most important preventive measure is the effective use of the toothbrush. To date only the mechanical action of the brush has been regularly shown to remove the bacterial and other deposits. Once gingivitis does occur it becomes easier to motivate the patient because then the ill effects of bacterial accumulation on the teeth can be demonstrated. The use of disclosing solutions shows up the plaque, and the associated areas of inflamed gum can then be pointed out. Thus the patient will have a reason for wanting to brush effectively if the relationship between the plaque and the inflammation is understood. It is a matter for regret that our efforts before the onset of disease are not so successful.

In the present concentration on plaque and plaque control the role of careful scaling is regrettably being minimized. Calculus, whether it is supragingival or subgingival, is the supreme plaque retainer. If calculus is not removed the success of any brushing instruction is prejudiced. It is also unfair to expect the patient to carry out home care procedures which are always quite difficult for some if the teeth are left in a roughened state either through lack of polishing or because calculus still remains. This is not to say that we should not begin brushing instruction from the first oral hygiene visit. But we should also at the same time help the patient in our way by beginning to clean and polish the surfaces of all teeth. Thus careful scaling is a most important factor in the prevention of periodontal disease. It is also a factor in the maintenance of the treated case. No matter how well we teach our patients to carry out plaque elimination procedures most will still form calculus in some regions and will require regular thorough scaling.

Attention must be paid to other causes of plaque accumulation. These are factors which should be dealt with by the dentist when possible; otherwise special methods may be required to be taught to the patient. Some of these causes (e.g. filling overhangs) are listed in Chapter 3 (p. 27).

Many of these conditions are discovered only by careful examination. The regular sensible use of X-rays is important and it is again emphasized here that the newer methods of panoramic mouth surveys are becoming increasingly important.

It has been shown that some plaque components may act as antigens stimulating antibody reactions in the gingivae with the effect of enhancing the inflammatory effect of the plaque. The mechanism of action has been extensively studied but is still not perfectly clear. However, our knowledge of this immune reaction would not appear to have any bearing yet on the type of treatment which we employ.

PERIODONTAL DISEASE

The approach to periodontal treatment may be outlined as follows:
1. Awareness by the dentist and the periodontist of the problem.
2. Informing the patient.
3. Awareness by the patient of the nature of the problem and the patient's reaction to this awareness.
4. Full diagnostic procedure, including detailed past and present medical and dental history. Diet and habit check;
5. Preliminary treatment planning discussion with the patient. Initial patient personality evaluation at this point.
   Assessment of degree of comprehension, i.e. patient's dental I.Q. and manual ability (e.g. arthritic?).
6. Initial therapy:
   Education, motivation and training in home-care methods, plus dentist's or hygienist's treatment of local factors.

7. Reassessment:

   Allocation:

   Patient co-operation good:

   a. No further active treatment necessary

   or

   b. Definitive completion treatment may now begin.

   Patient co-operation poor:

   Proceed no further, but may refer back for further training if thought desirable.

We should consider these points in detail:

1. *Awareness by the Dentist of the Periodontal Problem*

It is not the purpose here to go into this fully, but it has been frequently demonstrated that one of the main factors in tooth loss is the non-recognition of established periodontal disease by the regularly attended dentist. To be able to treat periodontal disease we must recognize its presence and preferably recognize it early.

2. *Informing the Patient*

It follows that the patient must be informed of the presence of disease and must be fully acquainted with the importance of dealing with it. If this is ignored the patient's fundamental role will be neglected. All too often patients present with advanced disease stating that years ago, when they complained of bleeding gums, they were told that they have 'a little gum trouble' and to—

   a. Use an oxygen liberating mouthwash (e.g. Bocasan, Amosan) daily, or

   b. Use an intermittent water pressure irrigation device (e.g. Water Pik), or

   c. 'You have pyorrhoea—nothing can be done. It's just a matter of hanging on until they have to be extracted. In the meantime, we will continue with your fillings.'

In spite of this the disease progresses. The patient has had no information of value because the dentist had none to give. Sometimes, however, the dentist has been well aware of the extent of the problem but has been too embarrassed to tell the patient that, in spite of regular 6-monthly check-ups for ten years, there now appears to be a state of advanced periodontal breakdown. It requires courage, but the extent of the problem should be explained quite clearly to the patient. *We must be careful in our communication with the patient to talk the same language.*

3. Awareness by the Patient

Once the patient is aware of the seriousness and extent of the problem there will be some early response, indicating whether there is a strong desire or otherwise to retain the remaining teeth. Often the awareness has been reinforced by some periodontal crisis, loss of a loose tooth, or recurrent periodontal abscesses.

4. and 5. *Full Diagnostic Procedures and Preliminary Planning Discussion*

It is beyond the scope of this work to deal with all the diagnostic procedures to be adopted. We are concerned here with those which may modify the treatment plans and the patient's ability to carry them out. It is important to assess the patient's attitude to dental treatment; is there a strong desire to retain the dentition, or would the work involved be a waste of time because the patient really wants complete dentures? A past dental history may reveal earlier attempts at periodontal treatment, gingivectomies and other surgical procedures. It should be of interest to hear the patient's account as to why they failed. Is the patient competent or willing to carry out home care procedures?

What should be noted are:

a. For most people appearances are important, so those who are untidy and pay little attention to their grooming are likely to be more difficult to persuade to spend time on their teeth (which are less visible).

b. Smoking is a factor in gingival disease, and heavy smoking, especially in the young, will prejudice or delay a successful outcome to periodontal therapy.

c. Alcoholics often make impossible subjects.

d. There may be a lack of the manual ability necessary to carry out the essential home care, e.g. the patient may be arthritic or otherwise handicapped. There may be a gag reflex, making the usual brushing procedure impossible.

e. Some patients on heavy drug therapy, for example phenytoin, may have difficulties in maintaining concentration except for very short periods.

f. With regard to diet, it has been demonstrated on a number of occasions that the nature of the diet has little effect as a cleansing agent and plaque remover. However, a high sucrose diet is plaque encouraging and the patient should be advised possibly to decrease the high consumption of sucrose. Some dentists may wish to carry out Snyder tests or modifications to reinforce this advice (*see* Section on Diet, p. 87).

g. *Habits.* These may include fingernail, pipe stem and thread biting, mouth breathing and tongue thrusting. 'Mouth-breathing' due to incomplete lip closure (*Fig.* 32*a*) will often lead to the development of an inflammation of the exposed gingivae (*Fig.* 32*b*) with the characteristic 'gum ridges'. It was customary to treat such a condition with the construction of an oral screen to be worn at night or, alternatively, the lips were sealed together with adhesive tape. This is rarely done today except that oral screens can be constructed for other conditions, but it has been shown that careful plaque removal before retiring at night will prevent the inflammation from developing.

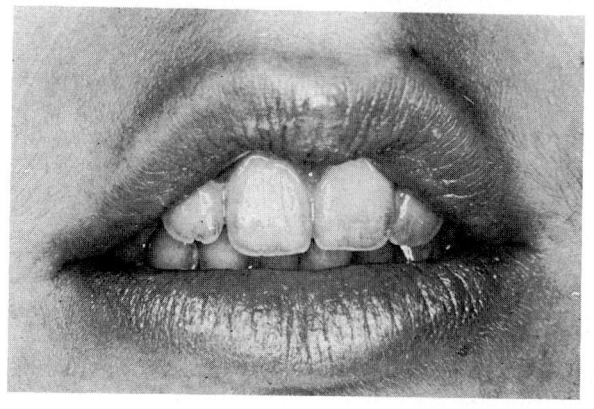

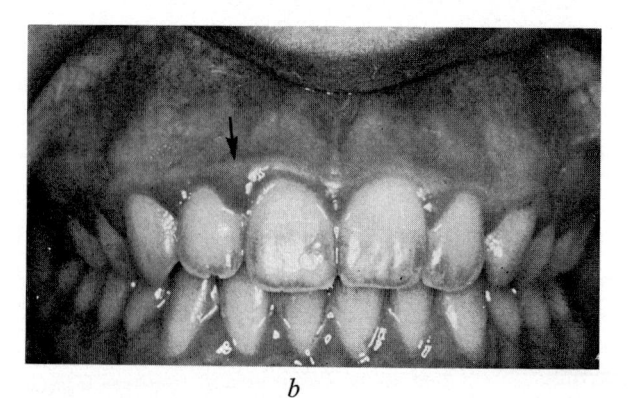

Fig. 32. *a*, Incomplete lip closure. *b*, Inflamed gingivae associated with incomplete lip closure. Note 'gum ridge' (arrowed).

CONTROL OF THE COMMON DENTAL DISEASES—PART 2

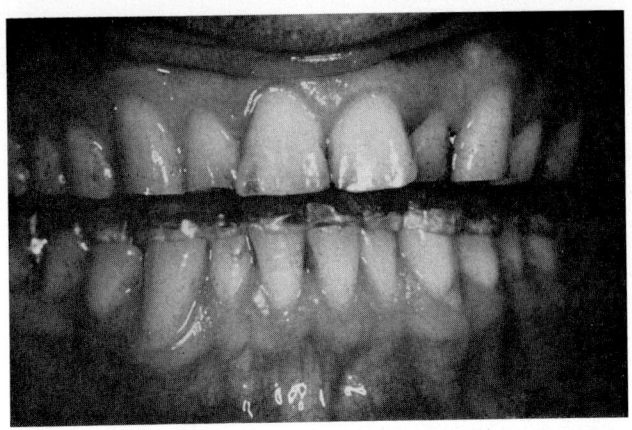

Fig. 33. An occlusal bite (or night) guard may be fitted where there is bruxism, or other grinding or clenching habits.

- *h. Parafunction.* Bruxism, clenching and 'lazy' mastication, or lack of masticatory ability (open bite) may all require correction. (*Fig.* 33).
- *i.* Deep overbite may initiate trauma to lower incisal or palatal gingiva. (*Fig.* 34.)
- *j.* Finally, and probably most important, attention should be paid to the patient's emotional state in that it may be the basis for much of the foregoing. It is also clear that many oral manifestations are totally or partially the result of emotional stress. Many workers for example have shown a close relationship between this and acute ulcerative gingivitis. And there is no doubt that conditions such as bruxism, clenching and biting habit often have an origin in stress situations and depression.

6. *Initial Therapy*

At this stage there may be referral to other members of the dental team specially trained to deal with these problems. A dental assistant trained as health educator may initiate the motivation and teaching plan of the programme. Audio-visual aids may be used, but these have very little or no effect unless they are used intelligently, with nearly always a one-to-one relationship with the teacher. Merely sending the patient into an audio-visual room with instruction to: 'watch this' is almost useless, as is filling the waiting room with a mass of pamphlets, booklets, exhortations to do this and that procedure. The teaching of mouth care is a personal one and each patient requires individual attention with a modified approach depending on all the personal idiosyncracies outlined above.

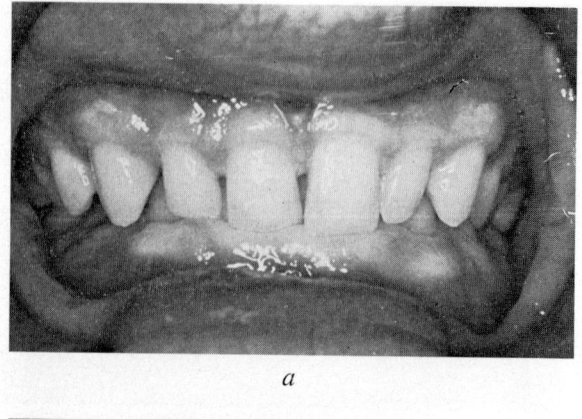

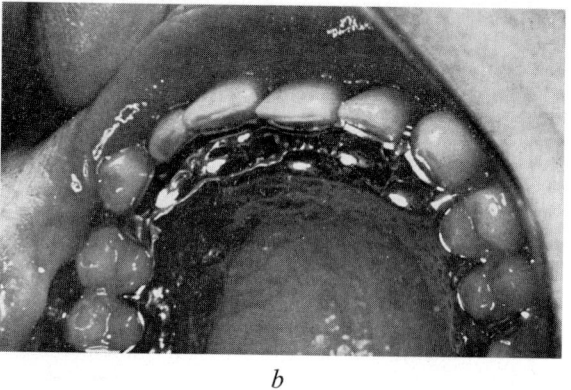

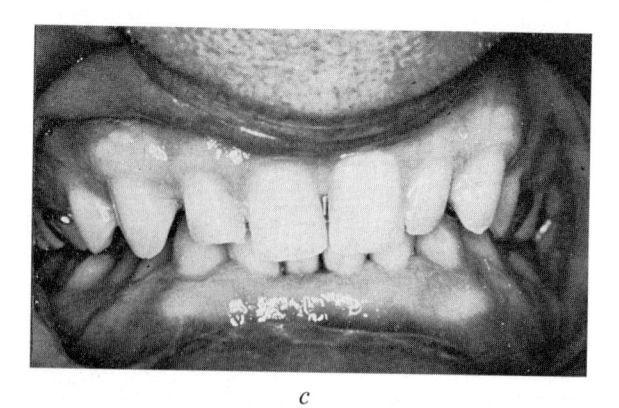

Fig. 34. *a,* Deep overbite with upper incisal edges traumatizing lower gingivae. *b,* The wearing of a metal bite plane. *c,* The improved overbite and protection of lower gingivae.

The early stage of dental health care training is often fraught with difficulties. If the dentist is not to carry this out himself, it is important that he does not just dismiss the patient with remarks such as, 'Miss Brown is now going to show you how to clean your teeth'. The response to this from a 60-year-old may well be, 'I am not going to be shown how to brush my teeth at my age by a chit of a girl. Why, I've taught three generations how to brush.' It is the dentist's own responsibility before handing over the patient to assess the patient's brushing ability—one way is to use a disclosing agent and demonstrate the plaque in a mirror held by the patient, emphasizing that however well the patient brushed it was impossible to deal with this invisible coating of bacteria until now, and that specific techniques will be demonstrated. It can then be explained that the hygienist or other auxiliary has had very special training in dealing with these problems.

The patient is asked to bring the regularly used toothbrush for the first session with the hygienist or dentist for oral hygiene training. (It should be noted that the term oral hygiene *instruction* is not used.

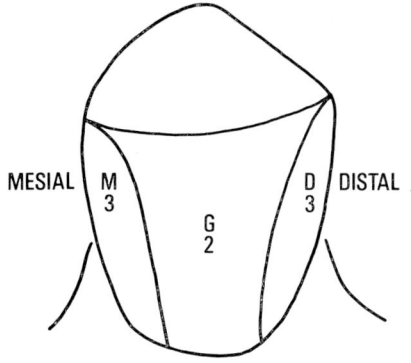

Fig. 35. Diagrams showing methods of scoring in making out a plaque index. Higher scores are given to areas where plaque is nearest to the gingival crevice and would therefore be more harmful.

The patient needs to be *trained* rather than just instructed.) It is pointed out that a new toothbrush should not be bought for this visit. We would like to see the old one in action. At this stage, the patient is asked to brush as if at home, leaving nothing out and taking just as much time as usual. It is useful here to set a stop-watch or timer unobtrusively and then to show the patient the brushing time. For most new and uninstructed patients the average time has been found to be around 25 seconds. After the brushing has been completed, a disclosing solution is applied and the neglected areas are pointed out. (*See also* p. 47.)

A plaque index may be prepared and done routinely as teaching progresses (*Fig.* 35).

It is tempting at this stage to go straight on to the demonstration of brushing technique. It is important, however, to avoid giving the impression that we are ordering the patient to carry out a number of

a

b

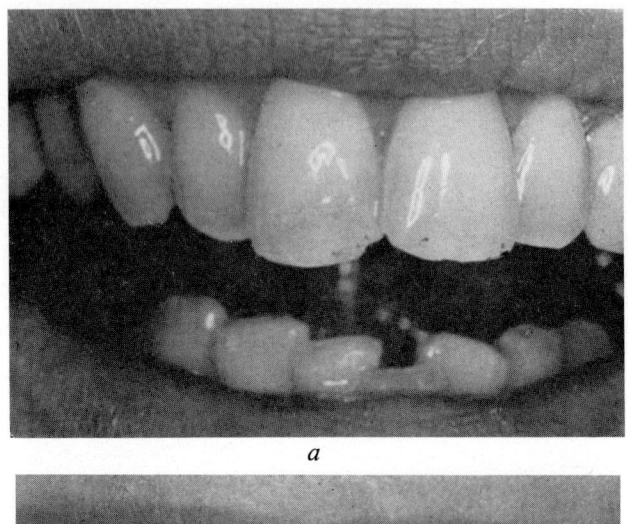

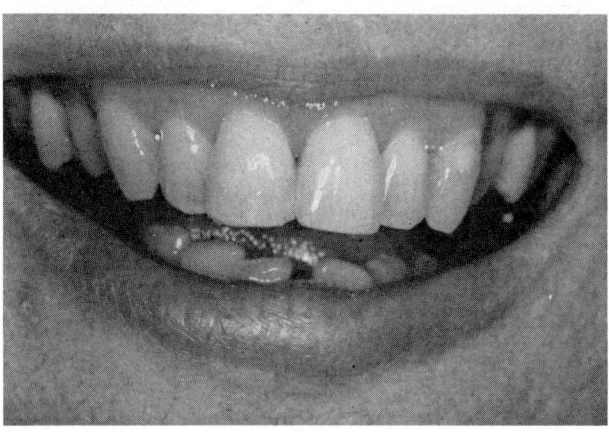

Fig. 36. Shortening or straightening incisors may take a few moments with a disc. The patient feels happier to brush her more pleasing teeth.

techniques without understanding. For this reason, some time is spent on describing the nature and the ill-effects of plaque and how it acts on the gum tissue and causes disease. Some colour slides may be used to demonstrate the beneficial effects of plaque removal carried out by other patients. Thus, brushing *technique* in our training

CONTROL OF THE COMMON DENTAL DISEASES—PART 2

programme assumes a role secondary to motivation and education of the patient. If the patient understands, he or she will want to carry out these procedures. Then it matters not what method is used, as long as the plaque is removed and the patient desires to remove it. We use the code M.E.D.A.R. for our training. This indicates *Motivation, Education, Demonstration, Assessment* and *Re-training*.

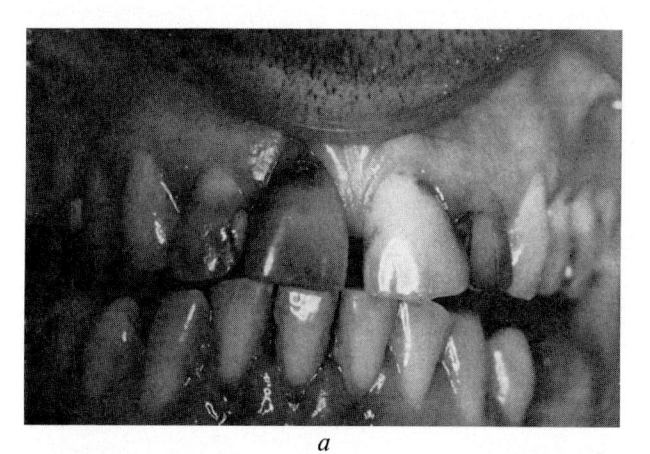

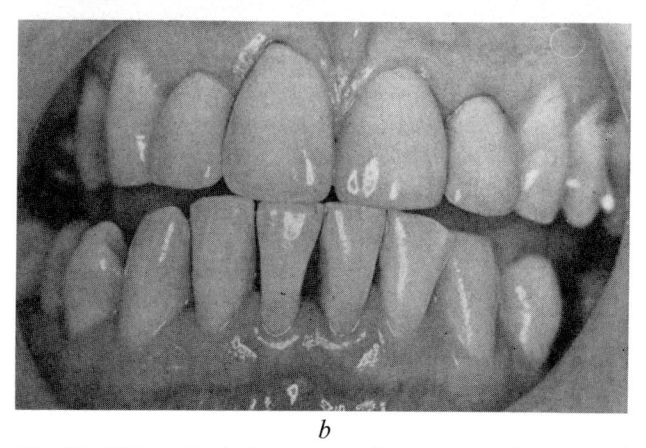

Fig. 37. This patient's home care efforts improved enormously following completion of his restorative work. Note the gingival condition, before and after.

Demonstration may be carried out initially on life-size models, but always ultimately the patient must be taught to use the brush effectively in his or her mouth, with suitable corrections by the hygienist or other teacher. There must never be any harsh criticism

PREVENTIVE DENTISTRY

such as 'You are very neglectful' or 'You are careless', but always encouragement.

Many patients often feel that their teeth are in a hopeless condition and that it is just a matter of time before they are lost, so why bother? This is especially the case if the anterior teeth are unsightly or the gums bleed excessively. A tremendous change in patient co-operation can occur after some reshaping of the incisors, replacing an unsightly anterior filling, or a couple of visits spent on removing gross calculus. The dramatic change may convince the patient that treatment is worth while. This again is part of motivation. (*Figs.* 36 *and* 37.)

a

b

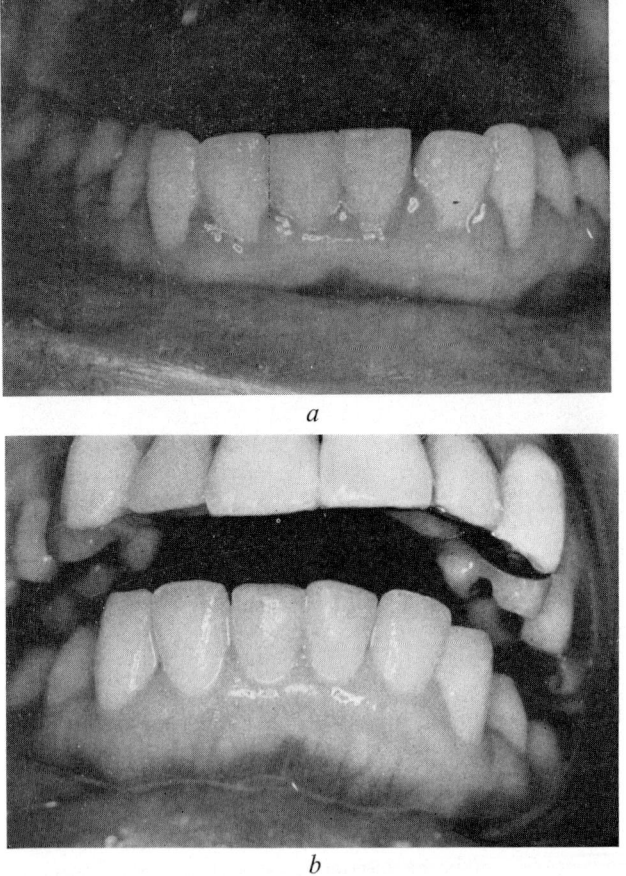

Fig. 38. This patient was taking high doses of Epanutin (Dilantin, phenytoin). It took one year of persevering toothbrush training (she could not use floss or other materials) to achieve the excellent result without surgery.

It is essential for the dentist to do all he can to make the patient's task easier.

It may well be entirely erroneous to persist with that timeworn injunction to brush after every meal. This encourages the patient to believe that the object of cleaning is food removal and leads both dentist and patient to ignore the dangers of plaque. Effective total plaque removal, which should be our goal, if carried out once per day is far better than two or three or even a dozen incomplete manipulations.

Kegeles (1963) has postulated that a four-point scheme should be adhered to where the patient is resistant to training and motivation or is having some difficulty. The patient should come to believe the following statements:

a. That he is susceptible to periodontal disease.
b. That periodontal disease is personally serious.
c. Periodontal therapy and plaque control are beneficial preventive steps to treat or correct the condition.
d. That the condition occurred due to natural causes and not as a punishment meted out by God for his past sins.

We may then go on to a demonstration of an effective toothbrushing method (not a *correct* method, but an *effective* method) and may be individually tailored to the patient's capabilities. There is no single method of toothbrushing adequate for all cases. Methods are described on pp. 42–47.

7. Reassessment

Perhaps 5 or 6 visits close together may be devoted to motivation and oral hygiene training. During, and at the termination of this phase it will become apparent that the patient is co-operating fully or not at all, with some in-between cases. If there has been full co-operation, the early stages of periodontal disease may have resolved and frequently, at the end of this phase, no further treatment except maintenance will be required.

There may be some patients who although co-operative, do not seem to be progressing satisfactorily or sufficiently rapidly and it becomes apparent that however assiduously they may brush, they do not eliminate sufficient plaque to resolve their gingival inflammation. These patients will require extra attention and possibly accessory aids in their home care. If there is sufficient loss of papillary height for the introduction of wood sticks of the Stimudents Interdens or Sanodents type, the use of these should be taught. They are almost always essential following the surgical phase of periodontal therapy, and patients will usually learn to use them quite readily. (*See* Chapter 3 for details of method.) The use of dental floss may be advised for others with difficult plaque removal problems where sticks are not suitable. Patients do not readily take to the floss habit and many give up after a time, however conscientiously they may have been trained in its use. The various flossing gadgets now being offered seem at first sight to be helpful but they have many disadvantages, principally that they tend to get foul during use. Adjustment of the floss in the holders is difficult and results in tangles and waste. It is often said that the patient who learns to handle these flossing gadgets must perforce have sufficient ability to use floss around the mouth without them!

Otherwise the use of interdental brushes or stimulators may be tried. Such instruments are the Perio-pak (Crescent) the Halex Interspace brush, the Wisdom Spacemaster brush. Patients vary in their likes and dislikes of these and on the whole the Interspace brush or the Spacemaster are the most acceptable.

Exceptionally, there will be some failures and serious consideration must be given to the termination of treatment at this point—some may be referred back for reconsideration of their problem and further motivation.

The few remaining patients who are completely unco-operative should be informed of the difficulties, and it is often best to set out the reasons tactfully in writing. A letter along the following lines is suggested:

Dear . . .

I am sure that you are aware that we have been very concerned about your dental condition and we have discussed the way in which your mouth can be restored to a healthy state. It has been emphasized that a great deal can be accomplished by your own efforts in daily attention to your mouth and gums using the methods which have been taught here. This is essential if your planned treatment is not to produce a poor result very soon after completion, and in that case you will probably be worse off than if the work had not been carried out.

We often have to spend 5 or 6 visits with a patient before the correct methods can be carried out at home and, as you know, we have been demonstrating this to you.

I am worried about the fact that for some reason you do not seem able to achieve as much success with our methods as we would both like. Obviously you would like to get on with the rest of the dental treatment as keenly as I would be to recommend it.

I therefore feel that we ought to have a discussion as to whether we can plan any changes in our approach, as you would not want to go to the trouble and expense of having dental work done which is doomed to eventual failure.

Yours sincerely

CONTROL OF THE COMMON DENTAL DISEASES—PART 2

Maintenance

This is a most important but frequently overlooked, part of periodontal therapy. It should have been impressed on the patient that there is a susceptibility to periodontal disease. Therefore, at the termination of definitive treatment, by which time the patient should be able to carry out all necessary home care procedures, an appointment for reappraisal should be made at an interval of 1 month. If there is good maintenance the appointment period may become 3 months, then 4 months, but unless the patient has developed an extremely good plaque control method the interval between maintenance recalls should rarely exceed this. A complete retraining is almost always necessary after a year or so.

A patient may say, 'I know I was due to come in months ago for a check-up, but I was waiting for your secretary to send me an appointment reminder, and as she didn't do it I didn't come in'. This demonstrates the dependence of some patients on external influences for their own welfare. Other patients are likely to be more forgetful about determining their own future.

We must all of us endeavour to lighten the patient's work load in controlling periodontal disease. It should be on the conscience of the profession that we have not yet discovered a means of treating periodontal disease which leaves the patient free to go about his daily living and forget all about us. This should be our aim. We should also not burden him with a mass of oral hygiene appliances, but prescribe the minimum necessary to ensure the simple maintenance of good oral health. It is salutary at this point to remember the report of the Editor of the *New Mexico Dental Journal* in which he says, '1972 has been the year of the great "control programme" boom, and reports are that gingivitis is down but suicides are up, presumably from frustrated flossers choosing the easy way out. We have promised salvation to the faithful, but have struck terror in the hearts of the arthritic and handicapped who cannot possibly pass the stain test'!

To Summarize

Prevention of periodontal disease involves the following:

1. Plaque prevention or elimination mainly and generally by brushing.
2. Careful inspection at regular intervals for the development of incipient gingival disease—probe gently for pockets.
3. Regular radiographic examination (*Fig.* 39).
4. Regular scaling and careful polishing. Most thorough scalings take more than one visit to complete. The number of visits is determined by the amount and toughness of the calculus and

PREVENTIVE DENTISTRY

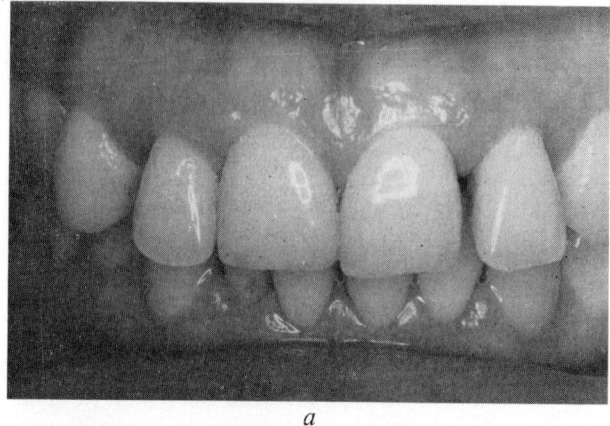

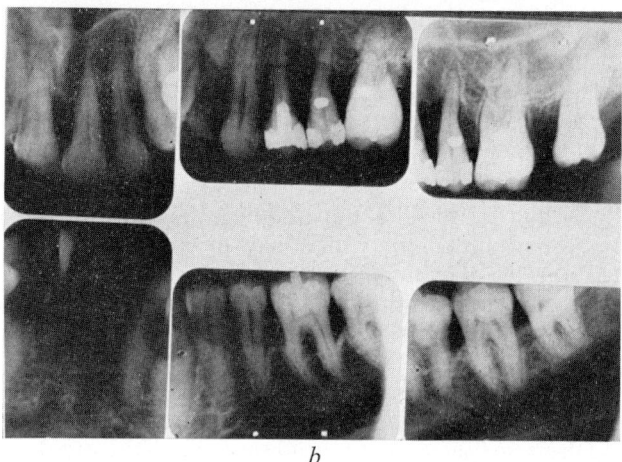

Fig. 39. The importance of regular radiographic investigation is shown here. The gingivae at casual examination appear to be healthy—pink, stippled, knife edge margins. The suspicious sign is the drifting lateral incisor. *b*, Radiographs reveal a disastrous situation.

coincidentally by the time taken for instruction and reinstruction of the patient's home care methods.
5. All our patients (almost without exception) will require retraining in brushing and other home care procedures after a year or less. Therefore we must check the patients' technique 'not by asking but by watching' at the regular check-up visits.
6. There should be a regular but simple recall system for all patients who have been and are under periodontal care.

7. Consideration of gingival health when carrying out restorative procedures (crowns, inlays, etc.). The crown margins should be supragingival where possible.

Conclusion

We can nearly always control gingivitis so as to prevent its progression to *periodontitis* and attain a return to a healthy gingival state. Our problem is that this requires constant vigilance and hard work from the patient and the dental team. Very few preventive measures will succeed on a community basis if we place the responsibility on the individual member of the public. Therefore what we must hope for is a periodontal equivalent of fluoride (especially water fluoridation) which reduces dental decay incidence without patient responsibility.

DIET AND DENTAL DISEASE

The difference between nutrition and diet should be appreciated. On the whole the population of this country does not suffer from nutritional disorders in the same way as many of the populations of the underdeveloped countries.

For correct nutritional needs there should be a balanced intake of foods such as meat, fruit, vegetables, milk and bread. These, in reasonable rations will provide the protein, fat and carbohydrates plus the minerals and vitamins necessary for health. In describing someone as suffering from malnutrition it is not necessarily implied, although this is often inferred, that there is insufficient intake of food but that the nutritional process is awry, either by excessive or unbalanced intake.

If, however, there is concern regarding the patient's nutritional state, e.g. scurvy, then reference should be made to the patient's physician.

However, the dentist and his team should be concerned with the dietary balance and in particular with advice regarding carbohydrate intake. Plaque formation and hence caries and periodontal disease is considerably increased with high sucrose intakes. The patient should therefore be instructed on the bacterial origins of plaque and on how sucrose takes part in this formation in a number of ways, one of which is by providing nutrition for the bacteria.

The following advice which is probably of use only if often repeated—with explanations of the reasons behind the advice, should be offered:

1. Carbohydrate intake is usually excessive and should be reduced where possible. This will benefit teeth, prevent obesity and perhaps may even delay atherosclerosis.

2. For caries prevention it has been shown (the Vipeholm Study, 1954) that sugar intake restricted to mealtimes will produce a lower caries rate than if sugar is allowed in the form of in-between snacks.

3. Thus emphasis should be placed on the perils of frequency of intake over the 24-hour period being worse (other than from a systemic viewpoint) than the quantity of carbohydrate intake.

4. Substitution of savoury or fruity non-sugary snacks should be tried, especially with children, where it may be possible to avoid cultivation of a 'sweet tooth'. This occurred without doubt during and immediately following the second World War when sweet rationing was present in the U.K. and many children grew up without the daily obsessive desire for candy bars.

5. The type of sugar containing food which is consumed is important. Liquids would appear to be less harmful than sticky substances which adhere to the tooth surface and there is some evidence that chocolate may be less harmful than, say, toffee. To advise one over the other would appear to interfere with the total philosophy of prevention which is that sucrose is harmful and therefore to discuss marginal differences may not be a rational approach.

It should be noted that 'natural sweeteners' such as honey and many fruit sugars may be equally as cariogenic as sucrose and indeed honey has been shown to contain high sucrose additives.

The 'hidden sugars' are a problem and sometimes these are protected by the apparent health promoting environment of the chemist's shop. It would appear that perhaps unwittingly the chemist supplies as much or more harmful cariogenic substances than the sweetshop. More harmful because most of those buying sweets in the usual way realize that the sucrose content causes dental decay. However in the chemist shop there are:

1. Baby foods—sweetened with either sucrose or artificial sweeteners.
2. Vitamin syrups—with enormous sugar content.
3. Cough drops and lozenges (up to 70 per cent sucrose).
4. Cough syrups (up to 44 per cent sucrose).
5. Chewable tablets of various types, e.g. vitamin tablets, antacid tablets (up to 55 per cent sucrose).

Patients should be told of the dangers of sugar in all these products and that the possession of a medicated or peppermint flavour as in cough or throat lozenges, or white mints is no indication that they are not harmful to the teeth. The label usually gives an indication of the sugar (sucrose, dextrose or other derivative) content and if more than 5 per cent is indicated an alternative 'remedy' should be sought. (Fujii, 1979.)

REFERENCES

Fujii D. (1979) Hidden sugar: O.T.C's add to tooth decay. *Am. Pharm.* NS 19 (11), 39–40.

Glickman I. (1972) *Clinical Periodontology*. Philadelphia, Saunders, pp. 443–474.

Goldman H. M. and Cohen D. W. (1973) *Periodontal Therapy*, 5th ed. London, Kimpton, pp. 427–461.

Grant, D. A., Stern I. B. and Everett F. G. (1972) *Orban's Periodontics*, 4th ed. London, Kimpton, pp. 363–410.

Gustaffson B. E., Quensel C. E. et al. (1954) The Vipeholm Dental Caries Study. The effect of different levels of carbohydrate intake on caries activity in 463 individuals observed for five years. *Acta Odontol. Scand.* **11**, 232–364.

Kegeles S. S. (1963) Some motives for seeking preventive dental care. *J. Am. Dent. Assoc.* **67**, 92.

Nizel A. E. (1972) *Nutrition in Preventive Dentistry. Science and Practice.* Philadelphia, Saunders.

CHAPTER 6

THE MOTHER AND CHILD

PREGNANCY

IT IS a common belief that every pregnancy invites the loss of a tooth by the mother (and some old wive's tales even include the father as a victim!). Pregnancy has no direct causation on tooth loss, but there are a number of factors which influence the rapidity and progression of incipient or already well established oral disease.

The expectant mother may be involved in a multitude of extra activities (apart from perhaps continuing in her employment as breadwinner) and these may include regular attendances at antenatal clinic, purchasing, making and otherwise acquiring baby clothes and preparing the home for the new arrival. Thus during this time her own oral care may be neglected, both with regard to home care and also visits to the dentist. There may be a change in eating habits with frequently an increased intake in carbohydrates, including sweets and candies. This may coincide with a desire for bizarre or exotic 'foods', sometimes to the exclusion of those with safer nutritional characteristics. Therefore there may well be more noticeable dental problems which are not directly due to the pregnancy, but to the associated self-neglect or to the extra attention which may be required during this phase. Thus there may be increased caries, especially at the gingival third of the crowns, and enhanced gingival inflammation.

The factors responsible for *dental caries* may be listed as follows:
1. *Diet.* The expectant mother may have her cravings for sugary drinks or sweets, or other cariogenic foods.
2. *Home Care.* This may be reduced for the reasons previously given and yet in view of the extra plaque which may form because of the increased sucrose intake, there should be more scrupulous brushing.
3. *Other Factors.* Acid attack in the plaque may be accelerated by acid from the stomach from nausea occurring early in some pregnancies.

Gingival disease can be quite significant during pregnancy. There are hormonal changes at this time, so that any mild inflammation (which otherwise may not be detected) may become quite marked sometimes with grossly enlarged and bleeding gingivae. Isolated enlargements may relate to the papillae of one or two teeth and these may interfere with eating because of bleeding. Although termed pregnancy 'tumours' these are composed of inflammatory tissue and should eventually resolve with the removal of the irritants, but occasionally surgery is required for complete return to normal. These conditions do not occur where there has been careful plaque control from the beginning. Therefore it is necessary to go over brushing and other home care methods with such patients and to stress the importance of paying particular attention to the regions where bleeding is experienced. It has been observed that where bleeding of the gingival margins occurs the toothbrush is kept away from that region. The patient must be encouraged to 'brave' the bleeding and brush carefully. Otherwise it may be expedient to advise the use of a cleaning cloth (a piece of thin towelling wrapped around an index finger) well rubbed around the gums and teeth of the affected regions.

PREVENTIVE ATTENTION FOR THE EXPECTANT MOTHER

The dentist should be attended as early as possible in the first stages of pregnancy for a thorough examination so that all necessary treatment can be carried out well in advance. Ideally he will refer the lady to the hygienist who should give instruction on maintaining oral health for mother and the baby. Advice should be given on a suitable diet to be adopted both to protect the parent and the developing child. Apart from the usual sensible mixed diet of carbohydrates, fats and proteins, essentially the mother's diet should include all the proteins, minerals and vitamins which the fetus needs:

An adequate daily intake of milk or milk products.
Proteins—meat, eggs, fish, poultry.
Vegetables—greens, cabbage, sprouts, etc. for vitamin A and iron.
Citrus fruits—oranges, lemons, grapefruit, etc. for vitamin C.

Now, it may be argued that the usual mixed dietary intake should provide all the above without necessary added requirements of vitamin C or vitamin A. This may be true, but in view of the sometimes remarkable changes in eating habits previously mentioned which are seen to be adopted by pregnant women, it is wise to discuss the basic vitamin requirements and how they are to be obtained, On the other hand there is still uncertainty regarding the need or advisability of recommending fluoride supplements in pregnancy. Murray (1976) stated that, 'Evidence with regard to the extent of placental transfer in humans has been conflicting', but on the whole it seems that the placenta may act as a partial barrier to fluoride. The amount of fluoride which is excreted in maternal human milk is very low (and this is true for cow's milk too). Because there would seem to be a regulatory mechanism in transfer of fluoride to fetus, it would seem that administration of extra doses of fluoride would not in general be advisable. The expectant mother should be careful to avoid taking tetracycline antibiotics; otherwise there would be a danger of discoloured teeth in the child.

THE NEW BABY

Breast feeding, if possible, of the newborn child is preferable to bottle feeding for the following reasons:

1. The maternal milk contains immune factors which have been acquired by the mother against various diseases so that the child has built-in resistance to such disease for the first few weeks of life.
2. The milk contains all the balanced nutrients.
3. The act of sucking on the breast is of importance to the proper development of the jaws. The action of the tongue and the pressure of the jaws and lips are enhanced by the effort made by the child to obtain the milk. All too often the bottles used do not give this pressure and the milk may be obtained too easily with resulting lack of stimulation of jaw growth. If, however, for some reason the mother finds it impossible to breast feed the baby, the bottle must be chosen from the number of well designed feeding bottles which simulate the action of the breast. The mother should be warned against purchasing a teat with a large hole or enlarging the existing hole with a pin in order to satisfy the impatient child. Too easy sucking may lead to 'tongue thrusting' and developmental errors.

Since little fluoride passes through the maternal milk, if the water supply is deficient, a supplement should be given to the child, starting at 2 or 3 weeks after birth. The dose must be worked out carefully according to the amount in the public water supply.

A number of cases of enamel fluorosis have been described and this has led to amendments to the recommended fluoride dosage according to age. (*Fig. 40.*)

Added fluoride dosage (milligrams per day)

Age	Concentration of fluoride in the drinking water (parts per million)		
	Less than 0·3	0·3–0·7	0·7 and over
2 weeks–2 yrs	0·25	0·0	0·0
2–3 yrs	0·50	0·25	0·0
3–16 yrs	1·00	0·50	0·0

THE MOTHER AND CHILD

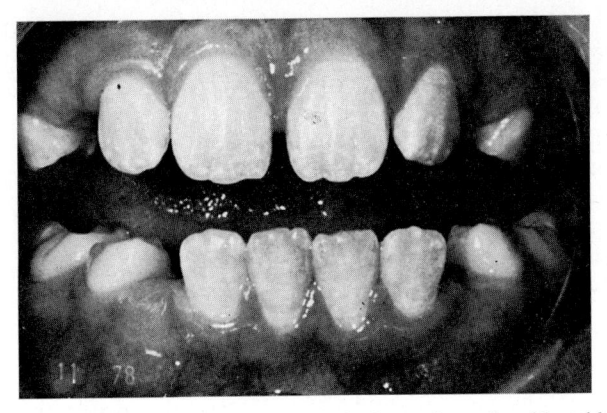

Fig. 40. Mild fluorosis following daily dose of one fluoride tablet (2·2 mg). (By kind permission of Dr J. Page.)

Sodium fluoride tablets (2·2 mg) contain 1·0 mg of fluoride. Therefore the smallest dose indicated above is ¼ tablet. Thus it may be better to recommend a fluoride solution specially formulated (e.g. Luride Oral Paediatric Drops) and which can be measured drop by drop more accurately than trying to break a small tablet into quarters. The bottles of fluoride solutions give the number of drops which equal a milligram of fluoride (in the above example 10 drops would be the maximum daily dose).

BABY BOTTLE CARIES
(OR 'NURSING BOTTLE MOUTH')

Some parents adopt the habit of giving the child a feeding bottle which is left in bed with the child all night. In order to make this attractive to the child the bottle is filled with water sweetened with sugar, or fruit juices or milk. The effect of this, when the teeth erupt at about six months, is the high probability of rampant caries characterized by initiation around the upper incisors and then eventually involving the deciduous molars. During the night, salivation is decreased and therefore its cleansing and diluting action in harmful acid formation is negligible. The child falls asleep while sucking on the bottle and the liquid pools around the upper front teeth and the warmth of the mouth enhances the bacterial proliferation and acid formation (Kroll and Stone, 1967). Milk, which in normal circumstances does not promote caries, becomes harmful when allowed to remain in the mouth for many hours. Therefore to avoid this problem the night time feeding bottle should be eliminated or at least it can be filled with plain water.

Small feeders of the Dinky type are similarly dangerous if filled with sugar water or fruit syrups. However, the use of the previously maligned dummy, or pacifier may be resorted to, but this must not be dipped in honey, jam or other sweet substances. A baby will suck something, often a thumb, a blanket or sheet. Massler (1963) says that after a satisfactory feed the child may still have a sucking need and that the dry nipple or pacifier is preferable to the comparatively hard finger or thumb and less likely to displace erupting teeth. The parents should be warned, however, against becoming too concerned about thumb sucking. Scolding, or even punishing a child will probably increase anxiety and lead to more sucking. Most will stop in good time. In any case incisor proclination due solely to thumb or finger sucking will be self-correcting after the habit is discontinued. Permanent protrusions probably relate to a skeletal tendency to a Class II malocclusion.

Many people believe that 'natural' sweetening substances such as honey are safe to use in feeding and mothers on being questioned about sugars and sweets for their child with rampant caries have vigorously denied their use. However, one often discovers that bottle teats or comforters have been dipped in honey. Shannon et al. (1979) show that honey is at least as cariogenic as sucrose and that the most frequent adulterant in honey is sucrose which is either added to the product or fed to the bees.

Cleaning baby's teeth should be commenced by the parent as soon as eruption commences. A clean cloth or a pad of gauze could be used initially, but soon a small toothbrush is employed and eventually the child should be allowed to handle the brush himself, although sufficient manual dexterity to accomplish a satisfactory cleaning job does not usually occur until about seven years old. Fluoride dentifrices should be used with just a small amount (about 6 mm) on the brush. As brushing is being carried out by the parent there is little danger of swallowing any significant quantity. The studies of Baxter (1980) and Glass et al. (1975) demonstrate that there is a wide safety margin in the low ingestion values of dentifrice found.

Weaning the child. One of the problems in the provision of solid (in fact minced) baby foods, is that many of these are purchased ready prepared in jars or cans. Examination of these—chicken, beef, vegetable, etc.—reveals that almost all are sweetened, some with sugar. The use of non-cariogenic sugar substitutes is no advantage because sweetened baby foods of whatever composition will almost always give the child a 'sweet tooth' or develop a craving for sweet things. The ideal plan is for the parent to prepare fresh foods and these are minced to a satisfactory consistency. If this is not possible careful selection should be made of the commercial brands and the

non-sweetened varieties chosen. What should be avoided in particular are:
1. Cola drinks.
2. Blackcurrant or rose-hip syrups
3. Sugary breakfast foods, e.g. Sugar Puffs, but even 'health foods', such as All Bran, contain quite significant amounts of sugar.

Medical and dental practitioners should refrain from prescribing tetracycline drugs, if at all possible, for children during the period of tooth formation and maturation, in order to avoid the dangers of unsightly tetracycline staining.

THE CHILD IN THE DENTAL PRACTICE

The relationship between dental practice and the child should be a happy one from the start. The earlier in the child's life that this relationship begins the easier it is to achieve. Thus ideally we should concentrate our efforts on instructing parents on the importance of bringing the pre-school child to the practice. The usual starting age for visits is $2\frac{1}{2}$–3 years. The advantages are many.

1. Very few children at this age will have been exposed to anxiety arising from tales of dental 'horrors'. It would be pleasant to believe that the public image of the dentist as a bloodthirsty sadist with forceps in hand and knee in chest tugging at a howling patient no longer exists, but regrettably almost all newspaper articles and other mass media publications tend to concentrate on key emotive words such as 'toothache', 'drill', 'blood', 'extractions'. The child who becomes a friend of the practice before coming under this harmful influence will later on reject these accounts of trauma as alien to itself and the practice. Indeed it becomes possible when the child is older to emphasize that the involvement in the preventive approach is one factor which avoids the discomforts which may have then been recounted to him by schoolmates.

2. It is more usual to find at, say, 3 years that any caries attack is minimal or non-existent (although there may be some startling exceptions) and hence very few children will have at this age associated their own teeth with pain. The dentist may therefore go on from this point maintaining a 'non-discomfort' approach for many years.

3. Attendance from pre-school age enhances the value of preventive techniques. There has been no time to acquire bad habits. Indoctrination can be slow and subtle and the child 'grows up with it'. The teeth are all fairly recently erupted into the oral cavity and the uptake of fluoride is enhanced. (*Fig.* 41.)

PREVENTIVE DENTISTRY

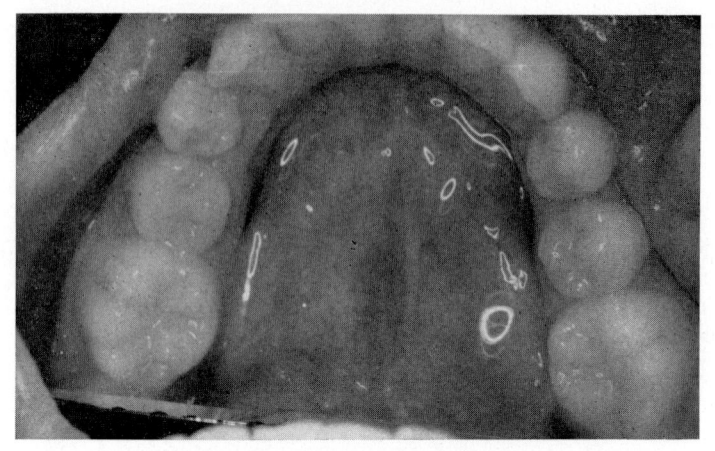

Fig. 41. A typical young adult who has had topical fluoride since the age of 2 years. He is one of a host of 20–30-year-olds in our practice who have never known what a dental bur feels like.

Some of the dental practitioners' attitudes which often still exist in relation to treatment of children should be discarded or modified. Many dentists still believe that:

1. Parents should be excluded from the 'treatment' room from the start, or as soon as possible, and that the dentist/child relationship is enhanced because of this and the dentist may then himself resolve the problem of cutting the necessary cavities in the teeth.
2. Gifts should not be given to children at the termination of the appointment. It has been said that this is a form of bribery and is therefore wrong.
3. Fillings should be done as soon as they are detected (as pin-point fillings) because it is relatively painless to drill the cavity form and it 'gets the child used to the drill'.

It is probable that these prohibitions existed because of the unpleasantness of repair dentistry and in order to enable the dentist to carry out his tasks in a calmer atmosphere. The change in attitude to a preventive one almost certainly means a reversal of these views:

1. It is necessary for a parent or responsible adult to be present with the pre-school child at the time of examination and possibly for some visits afterwards. We consider the parents (and we tell them so) to be members of the preventive team and therefore it is necessary to discuss with them the whole field of prevention in relation to their child. Thus at 3 years of age it is rarely possible for a child to grasp the techniques of brushing or the importance of

plaque control; neither can eating habits or the merits of food preparations be explained to anyone but a responsible adult. Other aspects of the child such as general health and physical or psychological problems would need to be known and recorded. A regular discussion regarding the child's progress is necessary.

2. Gifts are always given to our young patients unless something is done to affect our 'friendship' on a particular visit. The accusation of bribery does not apply because at no time is a child promised 'sit still and let me drill the tooth and you will get a present' because rarely is a tooth drilled. A gift is not 'earned' by submitting to trauma but is an expression of a happy relationship such as exists in one's family where gifts are given to sons and daughters because they are loved ones. An indication of this happy relationship is demonstrated by the frequency with which the children bring gifts for the dentist!

3. The presents for the youngest age group are nearly always useful in the sense that they are usually a balloon with a suitable inscribed dental message such as, 'Tommy Tooth says, "Take care of me, I'm hard to replace." '

THE FIRST VISIT

The young child is almost always welcomed by the hygienist who will seat the patient in the chair before the dentist enters and will demonstrate, often with a picture book, some aspect of the teeth. It might even be a children's story with reference to teeth. The dentist comes in at the point where the child is happily seated and may have had some sort of oral examination from the hygienist. A more detailed examination is carried out but very often without the use of a probe. A blunt plastic instrument may be used as some form of a seeker. For the few very apprehensive children the dentist may remove his usual surgeon's coat and approach the child in his 'ordinary clothes'. This gives him a more 'fatherly' appearance, but the occasions when this is necessary are rare. Even rarer are the occasions when the child will need to be examined seated on the lap of a parent in the dental chair, or even away from the dental chair at some more familiar easy chair.

A careful examination should be carried out as soon as it is practicable (it may not be at the first visit) and having due regard to the age of the child, the jaw relationship and development stages should be considered. It is important to look at the teeth in their closed 'centric' position. This is too easily forgotten in the occasional difficult situation of getting the child to 'open'! An OPG (or panoramic X-ray scan) is a very valuable diagnostic aid especially in the child patient, where very full information relating to the complete dentition, both erupted and non-erupted, can be obtained with the advantage that no films are placed in the child's mouth and the radiation dose is considerably reduced compared to conventional intra-oral methods.

It is always better to do some preventive treatment for the child, and most of them will accept a prophylaxis and topical fluoride from the first visit. It may be necessary with a minority to use only a rubber cup revolving slowly over the teeth (after demonstrating its effect on a finger nail).

RECALL VISITS

The parent of a child at school is asked to bring the child for attention at every long school vacation, i.e. at the Christmas, Easter and Summer vacations. This provides an interval of approximately 4 months between visits, giving 3 visits in a year. If, indeed, the parent is impressed with the responsibility of ensuring these regular visits, no recall programme will be required. Recall will, however, be necessary for pre-school children and those who are unable for some reason to attend in the normal vacation times or whose parents are unable to assume this responsibility. Ideally the mother who has been attending the practice as a patient herself will have received instructions regarding the dental health of her child from birth. There will be assessment of fluoride content of the local water supply—this information is readily obtainable from the water company concerned. Regrettably most supplies will be short of the optimum natural level of around 1 ppm and therefore some discussion usually takes place with the parent regarding provision by the mother of some separate fluoride intake for the child in order to make up for this deficiency. There are today a number of methods of achieving this: paediatric fluoride drops, dissolving F tabs in the child's drinking water, ingestion of tablets, fluoride and vitamin lozenges, etc., and in some countries fluoridated milk or salt. However, by and large most parents do not succeed in maintaining a satisfactory routine because it becomes demanding.

Instructions are given at a later date, i.e. as soon as tooth eruption starts, regarding initiation of brushing, and a suitable brush may be selected. The avoidance of the presence of food debris in contact with the teeth over long periods and the perils of sticky soothing syrups are emphasized.

As soon as the confidence of the child has been gained—and in the vast majority of cases this is on the first visit—a topical fluoride prophylaxis is carried out.

In our practice although many types of fluoride solutions and preparations have been used over the past years, as a matter of standard routine we use 10 per cent stannous fluoride solution (*see* p. 63).

THE EARLY CARIES LESION

At recall the young patient who has had a careful preventive programme will have little or no caries. However sometimes 'sticky' pits or fissures may be detected in recall or new patients. These should not be restored with conventional fillings. The effect of topical stannous fluoride applications should be noted over successive check ups and usually the incipient caries lesion will be found to have become brown and hard. If tempted to prepare a 'prophylactic cavity' the surface of the dentine is often found to be harder than expected (Massler, 1967). These sticky areas have been watched for many years and rarely has a filling been required.

RAMPANT CARIES

The new child patient that presents with rampant caries requires special attention. All too frequently there is a mass of amalgam fillings around the mouth with further carious breakdown of these already heavily filled teeth. Cervical decalcifications are frequently seen (*Fig.* 42). Deep carious lesions near, or involving, the pulp may be apparent. No 'permanent' fillings should be placed at this stage.

Treatment should take the following pattern:

1. Treat pain by suitable dressings, endodontic techniques, or extractions.

2. Other gross carious lesions are treated by excavating carious dentine and placing dressings usually of the reinforced zinc oxide eugenol type, sometimes with a metacresylacetate dressing sealed over any caries approaching too near the pulp and which has been left in situ.

3. The patient is taught plaque and debris control by careful demonstrations of its effective removal by brushing. A fluoride dentifrice is prescribed.

4. Stannous fluoride topical applications, as described previously.

5. Diet counselling, especially regarding carbohydrate and sucrose, is given to the parent.

6. Shallow cervical decalcifications—crumbly, chalky white areas usually—are treated by careful application of stannous fluoride solutions. They are not 'filled'.

7. The patient is brought back 2–3 weeks after the last dressing is placed, to check brushing ability and plaque control. At this stage a further topical application of stannous fluoride may be carried out.

At the next inspection, i.e. 4 months later, there should be some measure of control of the rampant caries. New cavities rarely will be seen. However, some already existing carious lesions involving

PREVENTIVE DENTISTRY

deeper layers of dentine may become apparent and these should be treated by excavation and dressings of the reinforced zinc oxide eugenol type.

Treated superficial caries will be seen to darken and harden indicating that remineralization has begun.

Wei et al. (1968) define the remineralization as a replacement of the 'lost calcium and phosphate with other minerals by chemical processes and exchange, substitution and physical and chemical bonding'. They further state that, 'based on radiographic and

a

b

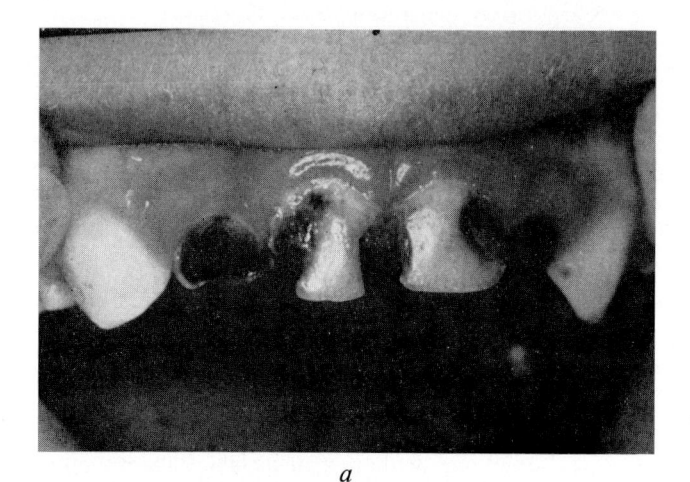

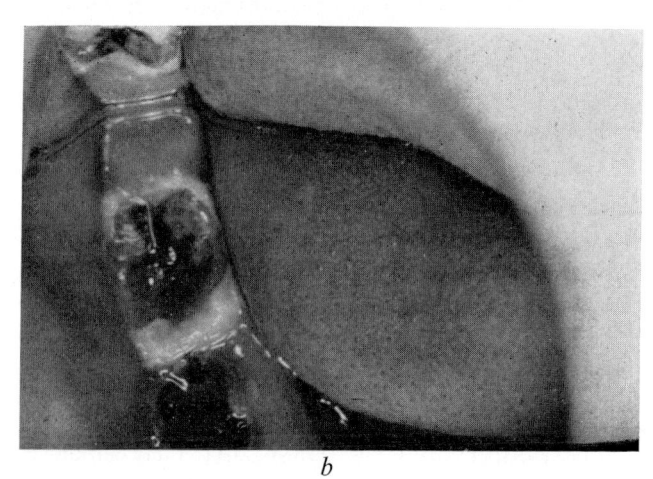

Fig. 42. Rampant caries associated with rose-hip syrups and sweetened comforters.

microradiographic evidence a 10 per cent stannous fluoride solution appears to remineralize carious dentine more rapidly and was superior to other remineralizing solutions'.

As soon as there is a dramatic diminution in new carious lesions permanent restorations may be placed in the 'controlled' mouth. Surface lesions such as the now brown cervical areas may be watched for years, however: eventually some may be restored with 'permanent' materials. Others may be left alone if the discoloration, which fades somewhat in time, is tolerable aesthetically.

It may take 2 years to gain *complete* control of a rampant caries patient but 'immediate' noticeable control is usually effected in 3–4 months. If no caries is discovered for three consecutive check-ups it is permissible to omit the topical fluoride and just gently polish all surfaces with fluoride-enriched paste.

Thus it can be seen that prevention of caries at the practice level does not consist merely of applying solutions of fluoride to the teeth. It requires a complete change in attitude and approach on the part of the dentist, the attitude of his patients by parent education, and of his staff which should be organized as a dental health team.

Basic requirements are these:

1. The dentist and his aides must be themselves convinced and confident of the efficacy of a preventive program. Assistants and patients will be influenced by the dentist's enthusiasm.

2. The 'prophylactic odontotomy' approach should be largely abandoned. Fillings and more fillings to prevent fillings does not make sense. There is evidence that the more fillings which patients receive, the more they require. A mouth in which the teeth are peppered with unsightly amalgam fillings on all surfaces has not had the best treatment although many dentists surprisingly consider that they are practising true prevention.

3. The dentist should re-think what constitutes a 'cavity'. Is initial caries attack a 'cavity'? The tendency is to consider that all breaches of surface should be filled. Thus the State dental service actually encourages the filling of 'sticky' pits and fissures, i.e. those teeth where a sharp probe will just 'stick'. This has been conventional teaching and it seems to be current teaching today. In a real preventive program 'sticky' fissures should not be subjected to cavity preparation and filling, but the effect of topical fluoride over a period should be noted.

4. Even in mouths where there are obviously many cavities requiring treatment this should be planned and action taken to minimize further cavity occurrence. Experience demonstrates to us all the futility of filling cavities in the rampant caries mouth. A

short time later there is another 'crop' of cavities. The rampant caries mouth is a special situation mouth, which Massler has called the 'caries infected mouth', and he has postulated control of the infection before embarking on extensive restorations (Massler, 1967).

5. The dentist must be careful not to be the causation of dental disease or recurrent disease. This may happen in the following ways:
- *a.* Inadequate preparations leading to further breakdown of weak enamel walls.
- *b.* Poor restorations leading to leaking and recurrent caries, and filling overhangs which may be influential in gingival problems.
- *c.* Over-enthusiastic polishing of teeth with brushes and pumice which scratch the surface and favour plaque attachment.
- *d.* Over-enthusiastic polishing of fillings which may overheat amalgam and affect its physical properties and also the use of abrasives may tend to lessen resistance to caries attack by removing the protective layer of enamel containing the most fluoride ion.

THE HANDICAPPED CHILD

Special consideration must be given to the handicapped child (or adult), although it should be borne in mind that more often than not the patient will not be as conscious of the handicap as the operator. However, handicapped patients require more time, thought and care in oral hygiene training and many of them will need more efficient plaque removal than their more fortunate contemporaries.

Distressingly there are too many different handicaps to list but we may consider the following categories:

Oral	Cleft palate, mucosal lesions, cleft lip, etc.
Heart	Congenital
	Rheumatic (acquired)
Senses	Blindness
	Deafness
Limbs	Arm movements defective
	Leg movements defective
Mental Defects	Continuous — retardation, emotional, psychic
	Periodic: Petit mal
	Grand mal

Generalized Systemic Diseases, e.g. leukaemia.

The dental team should evolve their own techniques for dealing with these main categories and should thus be prepared, and not have to devise anything but to modify the approach for the individual patient.

Oral Lesions

For the patient with cleft palate it is essential to use all preventive measures possible to preserve the remaining teeth. Efforts should be made to avoid extractions, as both deciduous and permanent teeth are needed for retention or stabilization of any appliances. Therefore appointments for preventive care should be frequent, and the intervals between recall should be short. Some parents initially may reject the deformity, and therefore avoid the necessary cleaning of the mouth. It may be that they fear doing harm to an area which appears to be already damaged. Thus, to avoid neglect for whatever reason, the patients must be told of the importance of home care and its bearing on future success. Later it will be necessary to demonstrate effective cleaning of any obturator or appliance.

Cleft lip is usually repaired at a very early stage and therefore presents little problem except that before repair there are feeding problems which require advice and assistance.

Congenital Heart Disease

Here exceptional oral hygiene control is imperative, with antibiotic cover for all procedures which might provoke bacteraemia. Increase of antibiotic dosage may be necessary during dentistry for those already on regular maintenance antibiotic therapy.

Rheumatic Heart Disease requires the same considerations as above, and these patients are more likely to be on permanent antibiotic cover. The risk for all these heart patients is, of course, the possibility of bacterial endocarditis. All septic areas (or potentially septic areas) should be removed under suitable chemotherapy cover.

The successful handling of these cases will depend on a careful history, records and a close co-operation with the patient's physician at all times.

Senses—Blindness and Deafness

The difficulty which must be overcome in teaching oral care methods, is of course, communication and demonstration.

The *deaf* will benefit by visual aids and carefully written instruction sheets for home reading. An intermediary who uses finger sign language may help to solve their communication problem.

The *blind*. Use of large tactile teaching aids such as models with large tooth brushes will help considerably. Cassette tapes may also be prepared and given for home use.

Defective Limb Movements

This calls for assistance of a third party or in lesser handicaps the use of various aids such as automatic brushes, patent floss holders, 'perio aids', may be tried, probably successively until one suitable for the patient is discovered.

Mental Handicaps

For those on phenytoin to control epileptic seizures it is essential to teach or somehow to ensure plaque control to avoid the tendency for gross enlargement of the gingivae. There is no doubt that this will not occur in the 100 per cent clean mouth (a difficult, often impossible achievement with anyone, but much more difficult with most epileptics).

Mentally retarded patients may require a great deal of patience to overcome fears of the dentist's environment. Therefore the approach must be gradual and in terms the patient can cope with. Restraint may have to be used occasionally and it is better not to use drugs. The brushing and other oral care may be best accomplished by nurses or other personnel if the patient is hospitalized. The value of preventive measures is soon appreciated in the growing confidence of the patient and the reduction in the amount of restorative work which may be traumatic for such patients.

Leukaemia

Careful oral cleansing with as much freedom from trauma as possible is essential with leukaemics; often antibiotic cover is required. No extraction should be carried out without very special precautions and it is better to refer the child to a hospital.

On the whole whatever other handicaps may be mentioned—cleft palate, diabetes, etc.—the main essentials will be the preservation of the teeth, the avoidance of major operative interference and hence primary prevention from the earliest possible moment in order to prevent the onset of destructive disease.

PREVENTIVE ASPECTS OF ORTHODONTICS

The general dental practitioner should be able to assess which cases of tooth irregularity come within his own capabilities of treatment. Other cases should be referred to an orthodontist either for advice only or for treatment as well. Trying to deal with situations beyond one's skill and diagnostic capability will lead to failure. Most of such cases are those in which abnormal skeletal patterns present. Cases in which there are localized irregularities or crowding respond well to the simple forms of treatment.

The dentist must be watchful of his young patients to check from say age 5 onwards the development of the arches and their relationship to each other. The size, shape and quality of the teeth must be taken into account because crowding which involves a genetically determined factor such as large teeth and small arches may involve some difficulty to resolve—it may not be accomplished solely by appliances, but on the other hand the timing of the dentist's involvement is important because later growth of the jaws may deal with the problem anyway. What the dentist must be careful of is subjecting a child to too early and therefore prolonged periods of sometimes unnecessary appliances and retention devices.

During his regular examinations of the child there should be careful recording of possibly harmful habits such as thumb sucking, lip habits, incorrect swallowing patterns, and possibly one could also include mouth breathing. Many of the deformities (such as anterior open bite associated with thumb and finger sucking) will correct themselves in time, if and when the child stops the habit,

a

b

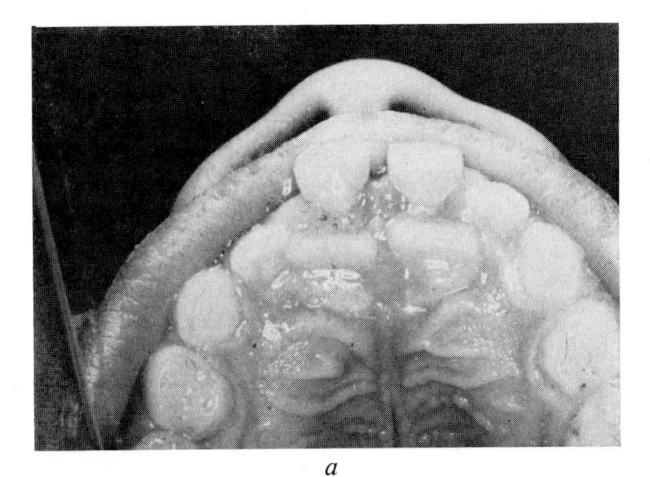

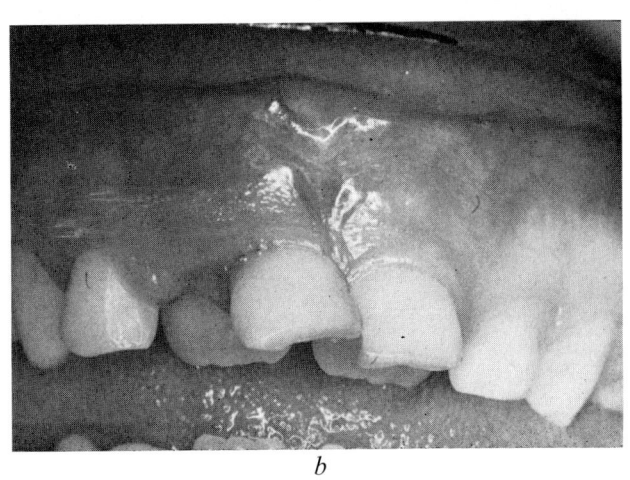

Fig. 43. Retained *A/A* causing malalignment of 1/1.

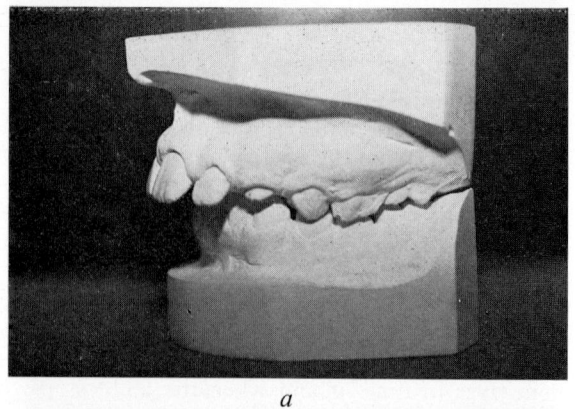

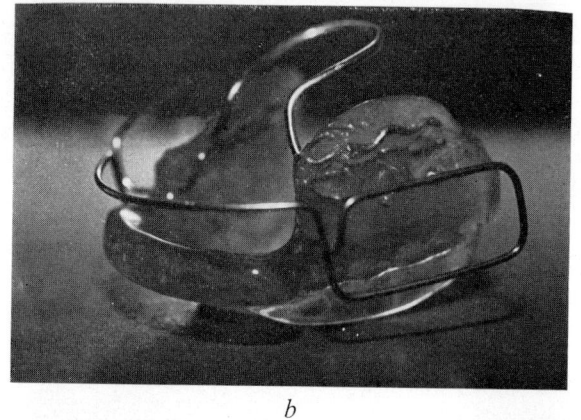

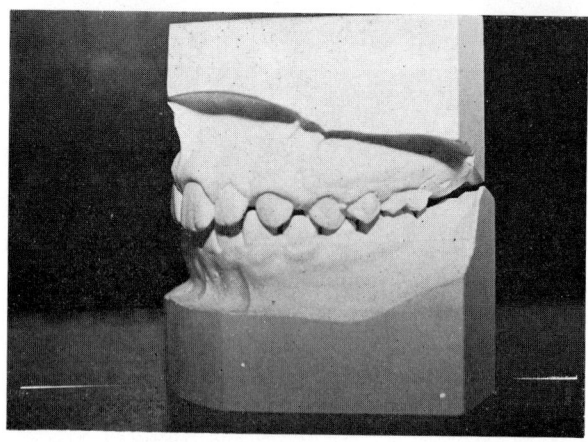

Fig. 44. Functional appliance (Bionator) used to correct a Class II abnormality. *a*, Relationship before treatment, *b*, Bionator, fitting upper and lower jaws, and *c*, After treatment. (By courtesy of Dr Alan Lynch.)

and therefore the dentist must here too be aware of the timing for interception. Many of these habits, if persisted in, call for much care, tact and ingenuity in therapy and often for considerable co-operation between dentist, parent and the physician.

The general dental practitioner should be able to deal with these problems quite simply with the use of a functional type of appliance, e.g. Andresen or Bionator described by Graber (1977).

The careful dentist who has prepared properly articulated study models will soon realize whether he is dealing with a Class II or Class III malrelationship. He would do well to refer these cases to a consultant orthodontist for advice and treatment. No orthodontic treatment should be embarked on without very careful consideration of the total arch relationships. However, the following may well be considered as being within the scope of preventive attention.

1. Retained deciduous teeth. The ankylosed tooth especially may cause malalignment of the permanent tooth and may also cause lack of development of the alveolar process (*Fig.* 43).

2. Poor restorative attention—loss of contacts due to caries or inadequately contoured fillings may lead to loss of space posteriorly.

3. Loss of deciduous posterior teeth may lead to encroachment on the space required for eruption of successional teeth (*Fig.* 45). Attention should be paid to the necessity for provision of a space maintainer but *careful* observation over a period may determine whether this is necessary, which is not always the case.

4. Crossbites in wholly deciduous arches usually do not require orthodontic interference as the permanent arches are not usually corrected by this early treatment. But where permanent teeth, e.g. first molars, and later, premolars, have erupted, crossbites may be dealt with by use of a removable appliance with expansion screw. Developing Class II relationships and open anterior bites may also be treated at this stage by a functional appliance such as the Bionator (*Fig.* 44).

5. Unerupted or erupted supernumerary teeth may cause malalignment (as in (1) above).

6. Individual teeth which are in incorrect labiolingual relationship with their opponents may be corrected by simple bite-plane appliances (i.e. they can be moved over the arch by a bite-raiser and palatal spring); once in the correct relationship no retention will be required.

The dentist must always be prepared to take further advice should there be any doubt, and certainly he must be fully conscious of the

PREVENTIVE DENTISTRY

consequences of the long-term effects of any extractions, whether serial or symmetrical and be especially careful when considering extraction of a crowded anterior tooth.

It is necessary to carry out careful radiographic examination of both jaws in order to record presence or absence of successional teeth and supernumeraries. A panoramic examination is the radiography of choice.

For details of methods and techniques the dentist is referred to one of the many excellent orthodontic texts especially intended for the general practitioner.

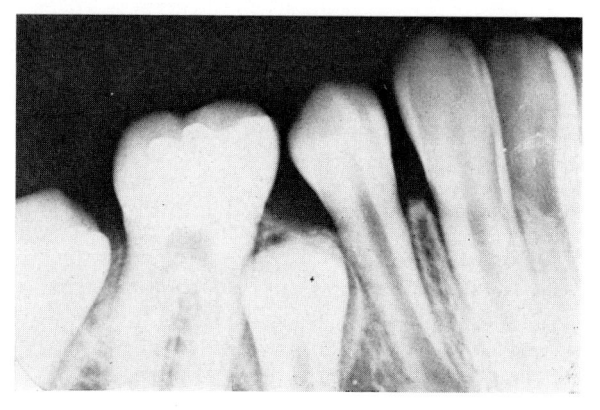

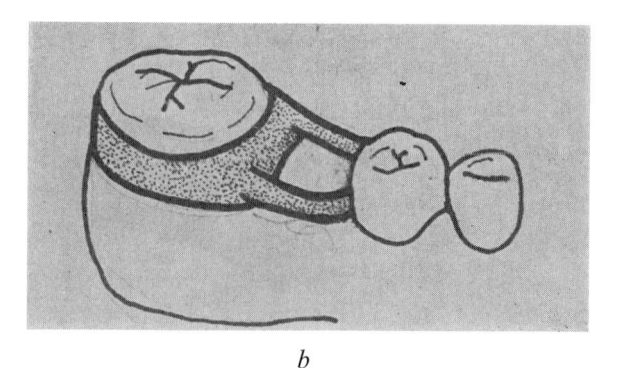

Fig. 45. *a*, Loss of a deciduous tooth with space encroached upon by first molar. *b*, A space maintainer would prevent this.

REFERENCES

Bass T. P. and Stephens C. D. (1977) *Basic Orthodontics for the Practitioner*. Epsom, A. E. Morgan Publications.

Baxter P. M. (1980) Toothpaste ingestion during toothbrushing by schoolchildren. *Br. Dent. J.* **148**, 125–128.

Dickson G. C. (1965) *Orthodontics in General Dental Practice*. London, Pitman.

Geiger A. and Hirschfeld L. (1974) *Minor Tooth Movement in General Practice*. St. Louis, Mosby.

Glass R. L., Peterson J. K., Zuckerman D. A. et al. (1975) Fluoride ingestion resulting from the use of a monofluorophosphate dentifrice by children. *Br. Dent. J.* **138**, 423–426.

Graber T. M. and Neumann B. (1977) *Removable Orthodontic Appliances*. Philadelphia, Saunders. pp. 229–246.

Kroll R. G. and Stone J. H. (1967) Nocturnal bottle feeding as a contributory cause of rampant caries in infant and young child. *J. Dent. Child.* **34 (6)**, 354–359.

Massler M. (1963) Oral habits: origin, evolution and current concepts in management. *Alpha, Omegan* **56**, 127–134.

Massler M. (1967) Changing concepts in the treatment of carious lesions. *Br. Dent. J.* **123**, 457.

Murray J. J. (1976) *Fluorides in Caries Prevention*. Bristol, Wright.

Shannon I. L., Edmonds E. J. and Madsen K. D. (1979) Cariogenicity of honey. *J. Dent. Child.* **46 (1)**, 29–33.

Tulley W. J. (1967) Prevention in orthodontics within the scope of the school programme. *Int. Dent. J.* **17**, 368–383.

Tulley W. J. and Campbell A. C. (1974) *A Manual of Practical Orthodontics*, 3rd ed. Bristol, Wright.

Walther D. P. (1967) *Orthodontic Notes*, 2nd ed. Bristol, Wright.

Wei S. H. Y., Kaqueler J. C. and Massler M. (1968) Remineralization of carious dentine. *J. Dent. Res.* **47**, 381.

CHAPTER 7

PREVENTIVE ASPECTS OF RESTORATIVE DENTISTRY

CURRENT views on restorative dentistry tend to support the broad general principles of G. V. Black (1908) but with some modifications. The original concept of extension for prevention was to ensure that the prepared cavity margins were placed in self-cleansing areas. In order to conserve tooth structure the preparation of class 2 cavities is extended only into 'cleansable areas', i.e. areas which are accessible to the toothbrush. Thus, in all cavity preparation the modifications are such as to avoid excessive tooth reduction. The ease with which tooth structure can be destroyed since the advent of the air-turbine handpiece calls for strict discipline and self control in its use.

In preparing proximal cavities it is essential to avoid damage to the contacting neighbouring tooth surface by being touched by the high speed bur. The placing of a metal matrix strip between the teeth during drilling will protect the intact surface, or it can be so arranged that the final break-through of the contact area is made with hand instruments. In restoring the same area it is important for the health of the soft tissues to ensure a naturally restored and well contoured proximal surface with good tight contact with the next tooth. The use of contoured matrix bands with suitably shaped wedges is essential for the above restorative procedures, and this applies not only to amalgam but is even more important in the anterior regions with the currently used composite filling materials where any 'flash' or overhangs are not only difficult to distinguish from tooth structure but are very troublesome to remove.

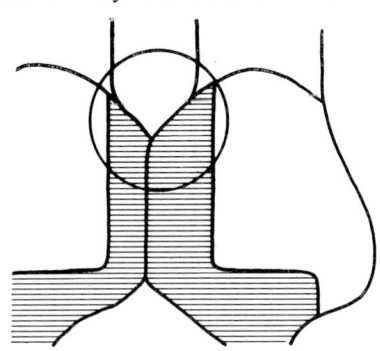

Fig. 46. A flattened contact area encourages food packing. A space opens up fairly rapidly between the teeth because of the wear between the flat surfaces.

A flattened contact area will close up the embrasure, which should normally be triangular in shape, and this will either crowd out any existing papilla, or will prevent accessibility to cleansing, and food will pack in from the occlusal (*Figs.* 46–48).

A well-restored marginal ridge will provide deflecting contours which will protect the interdental area.

If there is difficulty with amalgam in achieving a tight contact with the proximal tooth, consideration must be given to the use of a gold inlay. So far the experience with composite fillings in these situations is that the contacts become worn very rapidly, and it is doubtful whether there are any filled resin (composite) materials whose wear characteristics are acceptable enough to allow them to be used in Class 4 restorations.

It has been noted that occasionally some dentists, on failing to achieve a tight contact will open up the interdental area even more, in the belief that food will 'wash right through'. It is a poor remedy and rarely succeeds because it usually requires a separation of at least half a tooth in width and this amount of space will often result in tooth drift and loss of arch stability.

It is assumed that by now the dentist carrying out restorative procedures will be aware of the necessity of ensuring that the patient has previously been trained in plaque elimination methods. Therefore in crown or inlay construction the trend should be to prepare the margins supragingivally, as far as aesthetics will allow. Although it was taught for generations that in order to avoid recurrent caries the margins should be placed in the gingival sulcus or crevice, the disadvantage of gingival irritation, overhang problems, and possible operative damage to the attachment apparatus indicates avoidance of this situation as far as possible. If caries or other considerations necessitate preparation deep into the crevice care should be taken at the impression stage not to use destructive gingival retraction methods. Astringent cords or rings should be left in place for a few minutes only, and if electrosurgical methods are employed, strict precautions should be taken to avoid soft tissue or bone necrosis.

Much has been written about the importance of deflecting contours on the buccal and lingual surfaces of crowns, and the perils of not reproducing the ideal form. It is probable that there has been some over-statement, but the undercontoured crown with a flat surface may act as a plane for shedding food directly into the gingival crevice, and this may be harmful to the susceptible patient. Far more harmful is, as previously stated, the poorly contoured contact area. The size of artificial crowns and pontics is important, and in general they should be smaller in buccolingual width and in the amount of occlusal area compared to the natural teeth. (*Fig.* 49.)

Pontics in fixed bridgework should present a 'bullet nose' contact

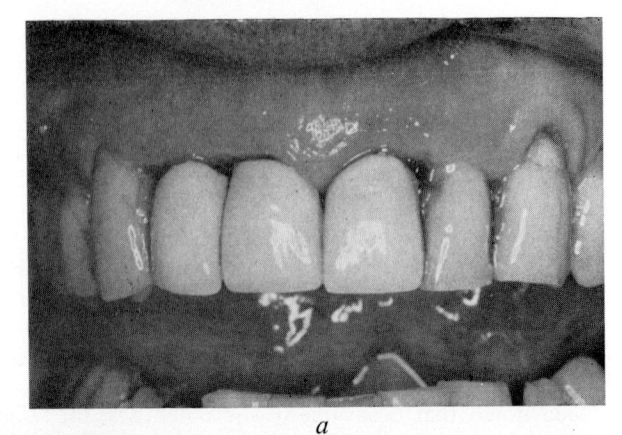

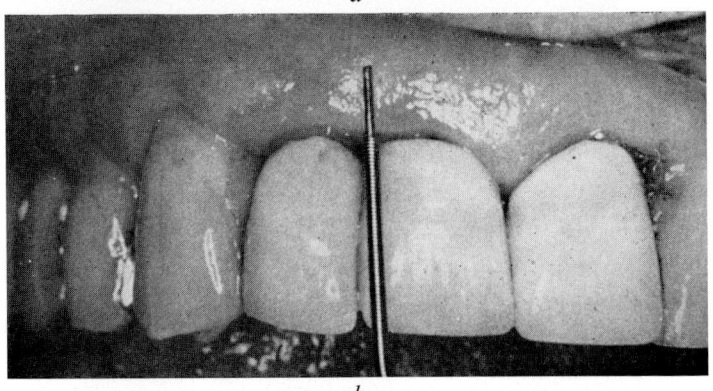

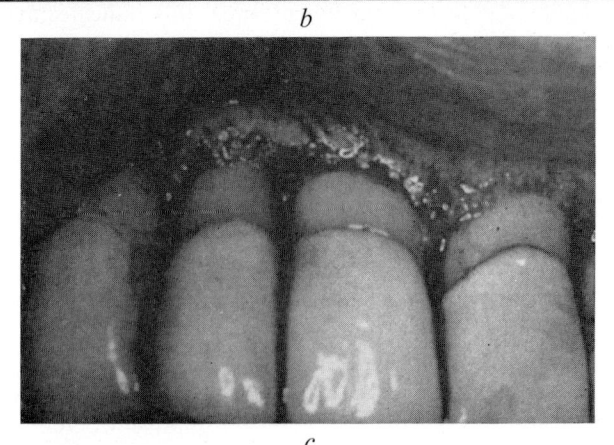

Fig. 47. Lack of adequate embrasure spaces has caused the deep pocketing and bone loss (*a*, *b*) The raised periodontal flap (*c*) shows the extent of the damage.

PREVENTIVE ASPECTS OF RESTORATIVE DENTISTRY

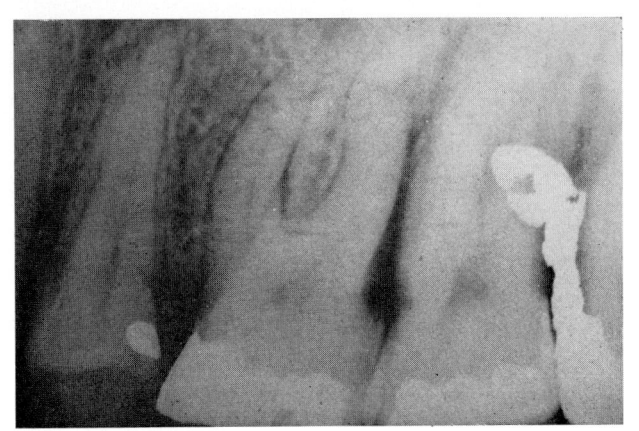

Fig. 48. The importance of a good well-contoured matrix band and wedges cannot be overstressed. Many teeth are imperilled by filling overhangs. This one must have been the result of exceptionally over-enthusiatic amalgam packing. The second molar was unsaveable.

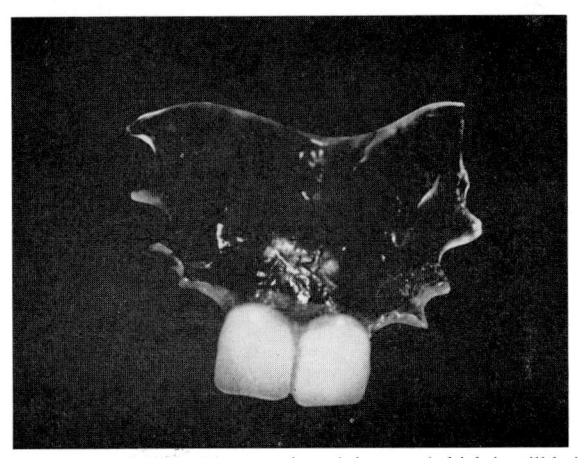

Fig. 49. The well-known 'gum-stripper' denture (which is still being made!). The sharp collets are mechanical irritants and the contoured gum fitted edges hold plaque against gingivae and teeth.

with the alveolar ridge, and the embrasures of the bridgework should be free. The patient should be instructed in daily cleaning, and some will need to be shown the use of floss threaders (such as Butler) in order to introduce the floss under any soldered contact points. The amount of effort and time that the patient will have to expend should be minimal and will depend on the care and thought which has gone into the design and construction of the restoration. The importance of good polishing techniques is described elsewhere.

PREVENTIVE DENTISTRY

In patients past middle age there may be episodes of rampant root caries. Casual examination of the crowns may miss these cavities which can extend rapidly and involve the pulp early. These may be in association with sweet eating in the old. Careful cavity preparation and filling, together with fluoride rinses should be undertaken. Saliva substitutes may also be prescribed for dry mouth.

All restorations eventually leak at the margins to a more or less extent and therefore there is no such thing as a 'preventive filling', However, preference should be given to those cements, lining agents, or restorative materials which contain fluorides, as there is

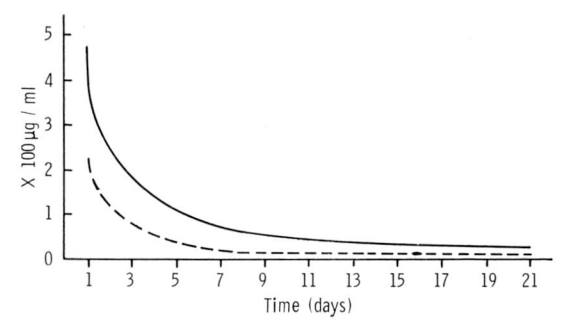

Fig. 50. Average amount of fluoride released daily from glass ionomer and silicate cement specimens. ——— Glass ionomer cement; – – – – Silicate cement. (By kind permission of Dr Ralph W. Phillips.)

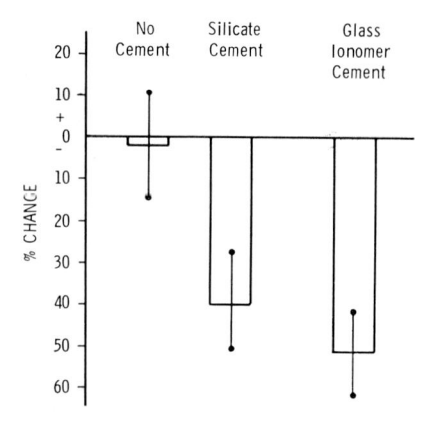

Fig. 51. Effect on solubility of enamel in acetic acid as influenced by two week's contact with glass ionomer and silicate cements. (By kind permission of Dr Ralph W. Phillips.)

evidence that they reduce the incidence of recurrent caries. (This was a notable finding with the fluoride-containing silicate fillings.)

Some polycarboxylate cements such as 'Poly F' contain fluoride which appears to improve the adhesive quality. However, there is evidence of fluoride effusion from these cements giving a combined anticaries effect. The glass ionomer cements which are offsprings of silicates and polycarboxylates seem to possess the desirable properties of these materials, i.e. the adhesive quality of the latter and the fluoride content and therefore possible anticaries activity of the former.

Maldonado et al. (1978) have reported on fluoride release from glass ionomer cements compared with silicate and showed a more than favourable difference in favour of the former (*Fig.* 50). There was also an effect of the glass ionomer cement on enamel solubility (*Fig.* 51). These findings are important, but the use of these cements require strict control and observation of mixing instructions and moisture regulation. It should also be noted that cavity varnish would interfere with the chelating effect (and therefore the adhesive properties) of these cements.

REFERENCES

Black G. V. (1908) *Operative Dentistry.* Chicago, Medical & Dental Publishing.

Burch J. G. (1971) Ten rules for developing crown contours in restorations. *Dent. Clin. North Am.* **15,** 611–618.

Going R. E. (1972) Microleakage around dental restorations: A summarising review. *J. Am. Dent. Assoc.* **84,** 1349.

Going R. E. (1972) Status report on cement bases, cavity liners, varnishes, primers and cleansers. *J. Am. Dent. Assoc.* **85,** 645–660.

Maldonado A., Swartz Marjorie L. and Phillips R. W. (1978) An in vitro study of certain properties of a glass ionomer cement. *J. Am. Dent. Assoc.* **96,** 785–791.

Marcum J. S. (1967) The effect of crown margin and depth upon gingival tissue. *J. Prosthet. Dent.* **17,** 479–487.

Skurow H. M. and Lytle J. D. (1971) The interproximal embrasure. *Dent. Clin. North Am.* **15,** 641–647.

Waerhaug J. and Zander H. A. (1957) Reaction of gingival tissues to self-curing acrylic restorations. *J. Am. Dent. Assoc.* **54,** 760.

CHAPTER 8

PREVENTIVE DENTISTRY AND SPORTS ACTIVITIES

INJURIES to the teeth and jaws occur in a variety of sporting activities and games. It should be a responsibility of the dental profession to advise on measures to cut down the rate of occurrence of these injuries and to take steps to protect any of their patients involved in risky sports, to minimize the dangers.

Two kinds of activities may be considered:
1. 'Contact' sports in which physical involvement between players is an essential element. Examples are rugby football, boxing, wrestling, and to a lesser extent soccer.
2. 'Individual' sports which may involve dangers. Examples are cycling, motor racing, cricket, baseball and swimming.

The dentist should determine whether any of his patients are likely to be involved in sporting activities likely to result in trauma to face or jaws and to assess whether any protection can be given.

In the U.S.A. it is mandatory for all schools to ensure that those engaged in contact sports are provided with mouth protectors in games such as American football. There would appear to be considerable controversy regarding the role to be played by dentists in relation to the fitting of mouth protectors, and in fact much of this work is done by the team trainer and is accepted by him as an extra source of income.

At the practice level it has been found that fractured teeth would appear to be associated most frequently with the non-contact sports. This may be due to the fact that with recognized dangerous activities such as boxing and rugby football there are usually facilities for dealing rapidly with injuries of all kinds, and fractured or avulsed teeth or jaw injuries are dealt with by immediate hospital referral. It is also probable that many of the players are already wearing mouth protectors. Fractured teeth have been reported most often from accidents arising in cricket, cycling and swimming. These are activities in which it is not reasonable to expect the wearing of mouth protectors for obvious reasons. The dentists' responsibility here is one of warning of possible dangers.

The provision of mouth protectors where feasible, i.e. in fairly short activities of a combative nature, have been demonstrably successful. The fabrication and design of a mouth protector should of course be considered in the same light as the motor car safety belt.

There should be an organized programme to ensure that the device is worn. Where school activities are involved, encouragement, or even enforcement, should be the responsibility of the school but the dentist should be aware of the problem and check that his patient is not exposed to an avoidable hazard through ignorance or neglect.

Mouth Protectors

They should be comfortable to wear, protect the teeth and the gingivae, and should not affect breathing or speech. Three types of mouth protectors are usually considered: (1) Stock prefabricated vinyl protectors; (2) Protectors with individual modification in the mouth; (3) Individually fabricated mouth protectors (*Fig.* 52).

Most protectors are made for the maxilla.

1. The stock mouth protector is usually supplied in three different sizes: small, medium and large. The appropriate size is chosen for each person and trimmed as necessary to fit on the upper jaw. Some remoulding in the mouth is possible by prior immersion in hot water. These protectors are generally considered to be unsatisfactory because they are loose and thus are not well tolerated. Also there would not necessarily be proper coverage of vulnerable areas.

2. Mouth formed protectors. These are usually supplied in a kit containing a plastic shell, often vinyl, which is matched to the upper arch and trimmed where necessary. The fitting surface is filled with a mixed soft acrylic or silicone and put to place on the maxillary teeth where the material is allowed to set while the teeth are gently closed together. Further trimming of the margins is carried out.

Disadvantages are the necessary excess bulk and therefore lack of comfort and interference with speech. The device is not easy to adjust for occlusion and therefore the wearer tends to chew through or tear it.

This method of protection is, however, reasonably quick and is less expensive than the custom-made protectors. One side-advantage is the possible use of these for fluoride application by filling the tooth side with phosphate fluoride gel and allowing the wearer to chew for four minutes. (This is of course of added benefit compared with those protectors less carefully adapted and which therefore can be reversed for either jaw, i.e. with the stock protectors.)

3. The protector made by a dentist, dental technician or a dental auxiliary to individual models is to be preferred. Stronger material—usually vinyl blanks—can be vacuum formed.

Advantages are careful coverage of vulnerable areas, lack of excessive bulk and the care which can be taken not to encroach too much on the free way space occlusally.

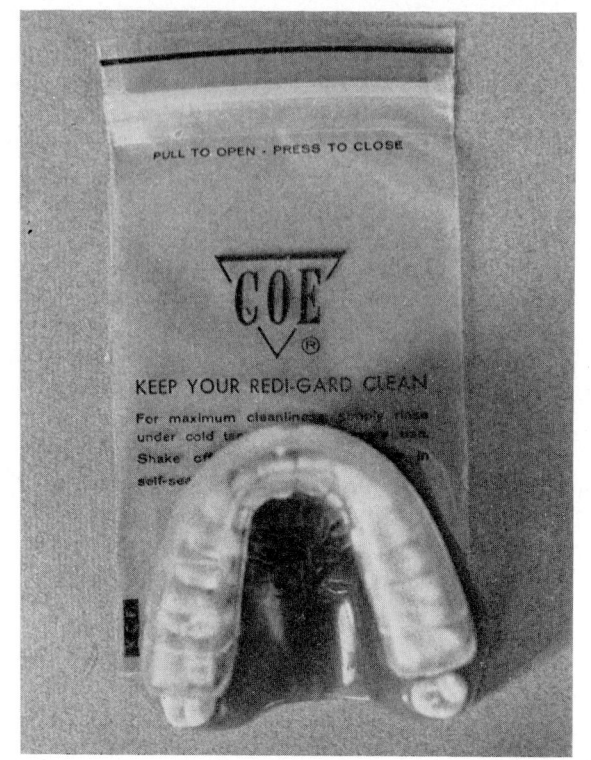

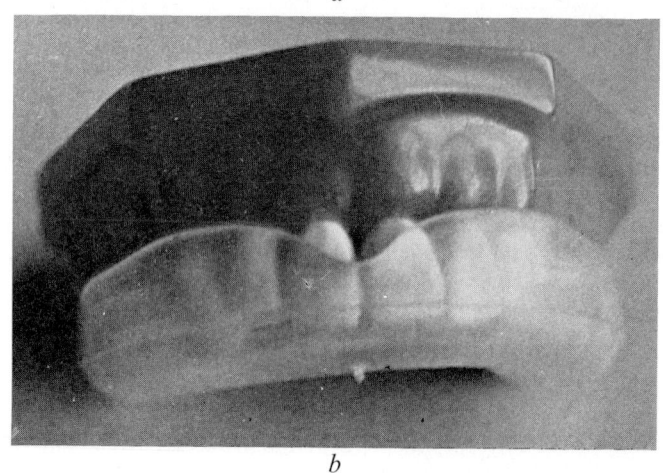

Fig. 52. Mouth protectors which may be remoulded and trimmed to fit the individual. Note the plastic bag for storing protector between games.

The protection of teeth and jaws, where possible by the use of mouth protectors, is a good exercise for the combined efforts of the dental team—in communication, advice and technique of fabrication. The hygienist should instruct in the care of the protector—careful cleaning after use and storage in a clean container.

Dentists who treat patients who have outstanding athletic distinction and who are likely to compete for honours in such gatherings as the Olympic Games must be aware that these patients may require special care. Often these athletes travel to distant countries and many cases have been cited where dental emergencies have interfered with, or cancelled, the athlete's performance. It is not sufficient merely to check for caries. A complete radiographic examination should be done (ideally with panoramic radiography), and the gingival condition should be evaluated. It is of the utmost importance to pay particular attention to the problem of partly erupted third molars. In these usually young patients, third molar periocoronitis would appear to be the main cause of emergencies and hence all doubtful third molars should be removed well before an important contest.

REFERENCES

Bureau of Dental Health Education and Bureau of Economic Research and Statistics (1964) Evaluation of mouth protectors used by high school football players. *J. Am. Dent. Assoc.* **68**, 430.

Cutler R. (1979) Focus on mouth guards. *Dent. Practice* **17** (March) 30.

Forrest J. O. (1969) The dental condition of Olympic Games contestants—a pilot study. *Dent. Pract. Dent. Rec.* **20**, 95.

Godwin W. C. and Craig R. G. (1968) Stress transmitted through mouth protectors *J. Am. Dent. Assoc.* **77**, 1316–1320.

Hertz W. D. (1968) Mouth protectors: a progress report. *J. Am. Dent. Assoc.* **77**, 632.

Stenger J. M., Lawson E. A., Wright J. M. et al. (1964) Mouthguards: protection against shock to head neck and teeth. *J. Am. Dent. Assoc.* **69**, 273.

APPENDIX 1

MATERIALS FOR USE IN THE PREVENTIVE PRACTICE

Demonstration Models and Teaching Materials

(For toothbrushing instruction and explanation of the structure of the teeth and supporting tissues.)

Information regarding these may be obtained from the Oral Hygiene Service, Hesketh House, Portman Square, London W1. Other audio-visual aids may be obtained from Messrs Nesor, London.

Toothbrushes

Wisdom Multituft, Medium
Wisdom 'Mouthmaster'
Wisdom 'Mouthmaster' Major
Oral-B 40
Oral-B 30
Junior
Gibbs Junior
Wisdom Junior
Wisdom 'Mouthmaster' Junior
Sensodyne Junior

Automatic Toothbrushes: Braun
                            Broxodent (mains).

Floss

Waxed (Johnson & Johnson; Boots)
Unwaxed (Johnson & Johnson, Oral B, Wisdom)
'Dentotape' (Johnson & Johnson). This is still probably the most acceptable floss. In spite of considerable pressure in favour of unwaxed floss there is little clinical evidence to suggest that its practical difficulties in use are compensated by any degree of superiority over conventional waxed floss. Superfloss.

Interdental Cleansers and 'Stimulators': Wooden Sticks
1. Stimudents (from U.S.A.).
2. Inter-dens (local pharmacy).
3. Sanodents.
4. Pick-a-Dents (plastic, U.S.A.; J. & S. Davis).

APPENDIX 1

Interdental Brushes and Tips

Interspace brush (Halex).
Perio-pak (Crescent).
Perio-aid (Butler).
Spacemaster brush (Wisdom).

Disclosing Solutions and Devices

'*Displaque*' (Pacemaker; Dental suppliers).
'*Disclosing Wafers*' Procter & Gamble.
'*Ceplac*' *Disclosing tablets* (Local pharmacy).
Rosepink food dye (Rayners; Food shops or Rayners, London).
Red Cote (Solution only) (Butler; Dental suppliers).
C Red solution (En De Kay; S. S. White).
Iodine-based solution (Iodine 1·6 g; KI 1·6 g; Water 13·4 ml; Glycerine to make 30 ml.)

Water Jet Irrigation Devices

Water Pik This is no longer on the accepted list of the Council on Dental Therapeutics of the American Dental Association (*see* pp. 31–32).

Fluorides

For Topical Application

Stannous fluoride crystals. (Oral Hygiene Products, 11 Approach Rd, London, SW20 8BA).
Various topical fluoride gels and solutions from the dental supply houses, e.g. from S. S. White (En De Kay), Luride, (Hoyt).
Applicator trays for APF gels. Various makes, e.g. Fluotray (En De Kay), Pascal, Hoyt.

Fluoride Prophylaxis Pastes

Fluoride prophylaxis paste (En De Kay).

Systemic and Local Fluoride Ingestion

Fluoraday lac tablets. 2·2 mg NaF. (Dental Health Promotion.)
Fluotabs. En De Kay. 2·2 mg NaF. (S. S. White.)
Fluodrops. En De Kay. 1·1 mg NaF in 0·3 ml=10 drops (S. S. White).
(Preferable for infants under 2 years of age.)
Luride Pediatric Solution (Hoyt).

Fluoride Rinses

Combined 0·4 per cent stable stannous fluoride and APF (Janar Inc., U.S.A., Johnson & Johnson).

Stancare. Tablets for stannous fluoride rinse 0·1 per cent solution (Block Drug Co.).

Fluoride Dentifrices

Acceptable from Colgate, Beechams, Procter & Gamble, Elida-Gibbs, or other manufacturers of similar repute.

Desensitizing Substances

For sensitive necks of teeth.

Emoform   } Europe }
Thermodent } U.S.A. } dentifrices
Sensodyne

These dentifrices are *not* intended for sore or inflamed gingivae. They should not be used for any soft tissue lesion.

As an application by the dentist or hygienist a paste of equal parts sodium fluoride, kaolin and glycerine is superior to all these dentifrices. The most satisfactory therapy for generalized cervical dentine sensitivity is a daily rinse for 10 days of 0·4 per cent stable stannous fluoride, glycerine and warm water (Iradicav, Johnson & Johnson).

Mouthwashes for General Use

Warm Water.

Normal Saline. 1·0 per cent NaCl in water.

Mouthwashes other than saline solution or warm water are rarely required and the use of peroxyborate solutions is likely on balance to do more harm than good.

Polishing Materials for use by the Dentist or Hygienist

For finishing and polishing restorations, and polishing the teeth after prophylaxis.

Contra-angle polishing head—snap-on or screw-in.
Small cup bristle brushes—snap-on or screw-in.
Rubber polishing cups—snap-on or screw-in.
Small rubber polishing wheels, screw mandrel.
Green and red rubber polishing cones—mounted.
Zirc Hygienist polishing strips.
Moyco extra-fine—narrow 2·5 mm cuttle strips.
3M composite discs 2 grits, fine/medium.
Zirconium silicate powder or paste.
Finishing burs—blunt, round and flame-shaped.
blunt, friction-grip, tapered fissure, carbide burs.

APPENDIX 1

Aids to Vision

1. *Surgi-spec telescopes* from Designs for Vision Inc., 120 E 23rd Street, New York, N.Y., 10010.
2. *Keeler telescopes* from Keeler Instruments Ltd., 21 Marylebone Lane, London, W1.

APPENDIX 2

SUMMARY OF PROCEDURE FOR PREVENTION OF CARIES AND PERIODONTAL DISEASE

THIS is essentially the procedure carried out to ensure that disease does not occur rather than the more usual treatment of already established disease, i.e. the causes are dealt with rather than the effects.

The dentist knows and makes the patient aware that plaque is very considerably involved in the causation of caries and periodontal disease.

The dentist explains to the patient the change of attitude from repair to prevention. This is related to the patient's present condition and past history of repeated or progressive disease.

The preventive methods advocated for the patient are outlined.

The hygienist may take over at the next stage and may carry out a series of preventive sessions during which the patient's plaque control ability is assessed and the patient is trained in the effective use of the toothbrush, possible use of dental floss and visits are continued until the patient can successfully perform the methods taught (usually 4 to 5 visits).

If we have to choose the most important single change which exemplifies today's preventive approach, it would not be plaque control methods, or fluoridation. It would be the realization that drilling a tooth is never a preventive measure but always a repair. Therefore cutting cavities must be done only when unavoidable, and when the previously described preparation has been completed.

The Child

Up to age 10. The mother or responsible adult should be taught the care of the child's mouth—with the child as interested listener. Topical fluorides are applied on a 4-monthly basis and a fluoride dentifrice is recommended.

1. Regular 4-monthly checks and prophylaxis after the patient has been rendered dentally healthy and is fully co-operating with oral hygiene.

2. At intervals of one year there should be a complete reappraisal and retraining if necessary in plaque control—brushing, floss, etc.

APPENDIX 2

3. It is customary in the U.K. to take 2 radiographs as caries check at roughly yearly intervals. Over the years this is *entirely inadequate* for complete diagnostic procedures, and for patients 'at risk'—through caries or periodontal disease—a full mouth study should be considered about every 3 years. A better alternative is a panoramic study (OPG—orthopantomograph or Panorex).

The current situation and the progress over the years—deterioration, improvement or static condition—should be discussed, with advice as to whether there should be changes made in the light of the new information.

After this the child or adolescent is taught separately but the parent may be called in to reinforce training at any stage. The parent is especially involved, however, in discussion of diet and the effects of sucrose, together with advice such as avoiding the consumption of sugary substances, but if sweets are given they should be associated with a mealtime and not throughout the day.

The use of topical anticaries agents is discussed with the parent and arrangements are made to make these applications every school holiday. Parents may be informed (depending on the dentist's arrangements) that the parents' responsibility will be to remember that school holiday means 'visit to the dentist', and therefore there will not be any recalls made.

A recommendation as to the type of toothbrush is made and an accepted fluoride dentifrice may be presented.

One great danger is to consider the preventive approach only in relation to *new* patients. The patient at risk is the regularly attending patient—year after year with never a really complete examination and assessment after the first one. It is too easy to become complacent about the regularly attending patient. The intervention of a third party, e.g. another dentist or hygienist with a fresh questioning eye, may often provide evidence and a warning that all is not well. There should therefore be a long-term care plan worked out for each patient with a programme such as previously outlined.

All 'old' patients require regular re-evaluation—new history, new thorough examination, especially for the presence of gingival pockets and mobility or drifting of teeth. Treatment should be formulated and revised if necessary, taking into account the patient's tissue response and attitude to dental care.

APPENDIX 3

SOME PRACTICAL PROBLEMS

AN extraordinary amount of physical change may often occur. Dietary habits may be altered—e.g. there are periods of lemon addiction with some patients, often associated with enamel erosion, or a previously heavy smoker gives up and perhaps starts to suck sugary mint tablets and a crop of cervical caries may result. An ageing patient may suffer from dry mouth, again with a greater tendency to caries. Thus the importance of constant vigilance with one's current patients is to be stressed.

In spite of careful preventive attention some patients will develop carious cavities. It is important, therefore never to promise '100 per cent freedom from the drill' a phrase often used by newspapers. Similarly we are unable to promise that periodontal disease will never occur. But our methods *will* diminish the incidence of these diseases to manageable proportions. We should not, therefore, have a sense of guilt because of the discovery of the occasional cavity or incipient periodontal lesion as long as patients have had all the care and vigilance which our preventive approach demands.

We must not accept an accusation of failure on these occasions from our patients. This can be avoided by previously telling them that we cannot promise total absence of disease.

An awkward situation may occur when one of our long-term preventive patients attends another practice for some reason (perhaps because of a move from the district). If the dentist is similarly enthusiastic about prevention all will be well. Sometimes, however, the new dentist belongs to the school of 'pit and fissure haters', who feel that all virgin pits and fissures ought to be drilled out if they are 'sticky'. (We might have been watching these 'sticky' fissures for years without deterioration in them.) The patient may be told that he or she *needs*, say, 6 fillings. The patient becomes understandably indignant at what is alleged to be the failure of our prevention. We have such patients who have received six or more tiny amalgam fillings barely into the dentine. It is necessary therefore to warn patients that such a situation may arise, and if there is any doubt to ask for a second opinion.

Where sealants have been placed into occlusal fissures it is not sufficient to note and replace any lost sealants. It may be that more damage may occur with some sealants which remain in position and which may be 'leaking'. All 'sealed' teeth should be carefully checked for such defects at regular intervals.

INDEX

Acidulated phosphate-fluoride (APF), 61, 64, 121
   applicators for, (*Fig.* 30), 64, 65
Aids to vision (*Fig.* 5), 12, 123
Alcoholics, periodontal prognosis, 75
Amalgam, finishing, 35
Appliances, orthodontic, (*Figs.* 15, 44, 45), 27, 107

Bass technique of brushing, 47
Behaviour patterns, 17, 18
Bitewing, 15, 125
Bridgework, 37, 111, 113
Brushes, automatic, 41, 42, 120
   B.S. (1979), 40
   choice of, 40–42, 120
   interdental, (*Figs.* 26, 27), 52
   method of use, (*Figs.* 20–22), 42–47, 79–81
Bruxism, (*Fig.* 33), 77

Calculus removal, 33, 34, 72, 73
Cancer, 9
Caries, diagnosis of, 4
   early, 99
   immune factors, 58
   incipient, (*Fig.* 3), 5
   'infected mouth', 102
   prevention of, 57–70, 99–102
   rampant, (*Fig.* 40), 99–101
   recurrent, (*Fig.* 2), 5, 6
   susceptibility to, 58, 75
Cements, 114, 115
Charters technique of brushing, 47
Child patient, 95–98, 102–104, 124
   and brushing (*see also* Fluorides), 69
Chlorhexidine, 20, 30
Communication with patient, 10
   on periodontal disease, 73–75, 124
Crowns in restoration, 111

Deafness, 102–3
Deep overbite (*Fig.* 34), 77, 78
Dental hygienists, 4, 6
Dental 'I.Q.', 12, 73
Dentifrices, 48, 122
Dentine, sensitivity of, 48, 49, 122
Dentures, polishing, 37
Dextranase, 3, 21
Diagnosis, 9, 75–77
Diagnostic aids, 12–16
Diet, 7, 87–88, 90, 91, 94, 99
Disclosing solutions (*Figs.* 10, 11), 23, 24, 25, 72, 122
   tablets (*see also* Plaque), 24

Embrasures, (*Figs.* 46, 47), 111, 112, 113
Enamel abrasion, 32, 33, 70
   dissolution, (*Fig.* 31), 70
   etching, 69
Epilepsy, 104
Examination, clinical, 9–15

Feeding the new baby, 92
Feeding bottles, dangers, 93, 94
Fillings, edges, (*Fig.* 48), 35, 36, 113
Fissure(s) sealants, 7, 58, 67, 68, 69
Floss, dental, 49, 51 (*Fig.* 23), 84
   demonstration of, (*Fig.* 24), 51
Fluoridation, of water supplies, 59
Fluorides, as primary preventive of caries, 57–69
   in cement, 36, 114, 115
   dentifrices, 48, 122
   milk, 66
   pregnancy, 66, 67
   prophylactic pastes, 122
   rinses, 66, 122
   silicate fillings, 114
   solutions or drops, 60, 93, 121
   tablets, 60, 93, 121
   topical, (*Fig.* 1), 5, 61–65, (*Figs.* 30, 41), 98, 99, 121
   (*see also* Acidulated phosphate-fluoride; Sodium fluoride; Stannous fluoride)
Fluorosis (*Fig.* 40), 92, 93

Gingival index, 27
Gingivitis, control of, (*Figs.* 9, 14), 21, 24 (*Figs.* 37, 38), 81, 82, 85
Glass ionomer cements, 114, 115
   as fissure sealants, 69
Gold inlay, 36, 111

Habits, 76, 105
Handicapped (*see also* Manual dexterity), 102–4
Hidden sugar, 88
Histories, medical, 11–12, 75

Interdental cleaners, (*Figs.* 27, 28), 52, 53, 54, 84, 121

Lemon juice erosion, 70 (*Fig.* 31)
Leukaemia, 102, 104
Lip incompetence, 76 (*Fig.* 32)
Long cone techniques (*see* Radiography)

INDEX

Maintenance, 85, 86, 87, 125
Manual dexterity in handicapped child, 103
 of patient, 75
Mentally handicapped, 104
Motivation, 21, 43, 82

National Health Service, 3

Oral awareness, 22, 23
Oral mucosa, 9
Orthodontics, preventive, 104–108
Orthopantomograph (OPG), (*Fig.* 7), 15

Parents, 96, 124, 125
Patient's record (*Fig.* 4), 11
Periodontal disease, 72
 initial therapy, 77
 home care, training, 79
 and restorative work, (*Figs.* 47, 48, 49), 111, 113
Phenytoin, 66, (*Fig.* 38)
Philosophy of preventive dentistry, 4–8
Plaklite, (*Fig.* 12), 25, 26
Plaque and caries, 49, 58, 61
 control of, 27, 29, 32
 disclosure of, (*Figs.* 10, 11, 12), 23–26, 79, 121
 formation of, 19
 index, (*Fig.* 35) 27, 80
Polishing, 32
Polishing cloths, 53
 materials, 36, 122
Pregnancy, 90
Probes, 14
 Svenska, (*Fig.* 6), 13, 14
 Williams, 14
Protectors in sports, (*Fig.* 52), 116–117, 118

Radiography, 15
 in children, 97–98, 125
 long cone, (*Fig.* 8), 16
 protection from radiation, (*Fig.* 8*a*), 15, 16
Reassessment, 17, 74, 85
Recall visits, 98
Remineralization, 63, 100
Restorative dentistry, 110–115
 and children, 101
 gingivae, 87
Roll technique of brushing, 44–47

Scaling, 33, 34, 72, 73
Smoking, 75
Snyder test, 58, 75
Sodium fluoride, 61, 62
Sports activities, 116–119
Stages in preventive dentistry, 9
Stannous fluoride, (*Fig.* 3), 62–64, 65, 98, 99, 101, 121
Stress situations, 77
Strip for polishing, 34, 36, 122
Sucrose and caries, 57, 58, 87, 88, 125
 and plaque, 19, 75

Teamwork, 5–7, 102
Tetracyclines and tooth staining, 95
Tongue, cleaning, (*Fig.* 29), 55
Treatment plan, 15, 16, 17, 18, 74–77

Uncooperative patient, 74, 84

Water irrigation devices, (*Fig.* 17), 31, 32, 121
Wood points, (*Fig.* 25), 51, 52

Zirconium silicate, 33, 34, 122